KW-000-634

CONTENTS

INTRODUCTION

A POPULAR American TV programme of the early 1960s began its narration with the dramatic recitative: 'There are eight million stories in the Naked City. . . .' In Great Britain, in 1975, there will be eight million people over the age of 65, if the 1949 Royal Commission on Population has estimated correctly. In simpler terms, this means that 1975 will see one retired person for every four of working age.

The African and Asian continents are beset with a mushrooming of their child and adult population which strains their food, drugs, educational and sanitary facilities and political resources. The Western world is oppositely bemused by its ever-increasing elderly population. The pattern in the United Kingdom resembles that in the United States, France and Sweden, where ten per cent of the population is over 65.

In Britain, the rise in the number and proportion of elderly people goes back to the actual birth-rate in the second half of the nineteenth century, which was so much higher than the present day, The survival rate of this population has improved immeasurably, owing firstly to Public Health measures and secondly to the introduction of the antibiotics. Such items as better sewage disposal, chlorination of tap water, vaccination and immunization programmes against smallpox and diphtheria, quarantine measures at ports and disinfection reduced the morbidity of local populations. The sulphonamide drugs and penicillin, streptomycin and the tetracycline antibiotics have eliminated the killer effect of scarlet fever, childbed fever, meningitis, tuberculosis and, to a large extent, pneumonia –

the previous 'captain of the men of death' for old people –
all on a national scale.

Yet while it is true that life expectancy at birth in 1967
is 67 years for a male and for a female 72 years, compared
with 1930 when it was 56 and 60 years for male and female
respectively, there has for the past century been little change
in life expectancy at 65. Confirmation of this is soon apparent, when an old age pensioner approaches a life insurance
office to negotiate a premium for a life policy commencing
in the seventh decade. Progress in medicine has clearly
benefited children and the middle-aged. Failure to influence
the degenerative diseases such as hardening of the arteries,
or to achieve greater control of tissue cancers, has meant
failure to increase the life expectancy of old people pro-
portionately.

Thus this increased section of the general population,
the elderly, will still have a considerable share of sickness
and infirmity. Most old people strive to remain physically
independent as long as possible, but some degree of dependence on relatives, friends and the community services is
invariable after the age of 80. This social factor is of much
greater significance when an old person becomes truly sick
or disabled, because then his or her chances of recovery
and return to community life depend on factors which the
doctor and his drugs alone may be unable to influence.

This book sets out to show how the medical profession,
faced with the indifference of the lay public and of doctors
and nurses in its own ranks towards the needs of the aged
sick, produced its own answer. The specialty of geriatrics
arose to seek out the medical and social problems of the
elderly sick, understand them and apply scientific and
humanitarian principles to solve them.

'AEGIS' AND THE BOOK *SANS EVERYTHING*

Since I began writing the manuscript for this book, Nelson have published the book *Sans Everything* by Barbara Robb for 'Aegis'. The letters stand for 'aid for the elderly in government institutions', a phrase which is presumed by the members of Aegis to be self-explanatory. I first heard about Aegis when I read C. H. Rolph's article in the *New Statesman* in February 1966 on the plight of old people in mental hospitals. He used the term 'geriatrics' in that article without defining it for his readers but generally equating it with the care of senile dementia and irremediable or incapacitating sickness in the elderly – a conception which I have discussed in the earlier part of this book. At the time I read the article, I considered sending a letter to the editor to point out to this journalist, whose favourite, and admirable, theme is the protection of citizens' liberties, that his article 'fell down' by failing to define geriatrics. I decided against writing as I felt it would be too difficult to define and polarize 'geriatrics' in a small space.

When I came to write the chapter on 'The meaning of geriatrics', I carefully considered mentioning Aegis in addition to the other societies and groups noted. This again was before the publication of *Sans Everything* which, as Aegis must have hoped it would, acted as powerful propaganda for its activities and a catalyst for 'shake-up' activity in the Ministry of Health, hospital management committees and mental and geriatric hospitals caring for the elderly. Prior to *Sans Everything* and the discussion of Project 70 in it, I was not aware that Aegis had evolved a constructive and analysed approach to the complex problems of the elderly that I have discussed at length in the present book.

Apart from its being a best-seller to the general public, I expect that most people working with or among the sick elderly in any hospital will have read *Sans Everything* and, like myself, have given it much reflection.

Whereas my own book sets out to discuss the advances and opportunities and successes in geriatric units, Miss Robb's sets out to show alleged cruelties and regressive practices and failures in mental hospitals caring for the elderly. It does not essay any definition of geriatrics along the lines indicated in my book. Its authors are obviously overridingly concerned with faults to be rectified, and getting this done quickly. I personally think, though, that to welcome their book unreservedly I should have to have been a medical practitioner in general wards accommodating the 'chronic sick', say, twenty years ago. As a picture of present-day care of the elderly it is one-sided. I hope *Later Life: Geriatrics Today and Tomorrow* may among other things redress the balance. There must be fifty anecdotes of success stories, warmth, kindness, help and rehabilitation of the elderly for every story of apathy, indifference, intolerance or viciousness published in *Sans*. All of us have met the petty dictatorial nurse or ward sister, the callous orderly and the indifferent doctor from time to time, and those of us with the power and the resolve have seen to it that these people are restricted or dismissed from their activities. I feel that loyal, hard-working and kind doctors and nurses must have felt hurt, however far this was from the intention, by the generalized accusations of their colleagues who contributed to the Aegis book.

But whether or not you agree with its method of presentation, Aegis has made its point and its originators must feel some satisfaction on this score. Barbara Robb admits in the book's preface that there is inadequate teaching of modern geriatrics in all sections of the National Health Service. I hope that my own book helps to correct this.

From time to time, all of us working in geriatric units feel frustrated by the slow progress of improvement in this or that section of ward or outpatient or day hospital development. We come up against the economic difficulties that bog down a National Health Service, tied by Exchequer red tape and the problems of determining segmental priorities; so that seeing a new piece of equipment at the Hospital Centre, for example, which could increase patients' rehabilitation, does not mean we can automatically order it for our department; or feeling that a showerbath would be a useful addition for bathing more disabled or frail patients does not signify that such new bathroom accommodation can be entered in next year's estimates. It is at moments or phases like these that many of us have felt like writing letters to our M.P.s or to the Sunday papers or even publishing a 'book of revelations' so that we could cut across the baulk.

Nevertheless we usually find that we can cool our tempers down by a backward glance. That is to say, we recall what things were like two and four and eight years ago when the whole 'movement' began – for the picture of this I refer you to the body of the first chapter – and then enumerate the positive changes and points of real progress that have very clearly been achieved. This comparison helps restore our equilibrium without reducing our firm resolve to go on improving the nursing and medical care of the elderly. The fact that we have gradually raised our baseline for such care helps guide our frustrations into the most constructive pathways.

1

THE MEANING OF GERIATRICS

THE CHRONIC SICK 'IMAGE'

WHEN doctors are looking around for a suitable name or title for an illness or a group of diseases, they generally do one of two things. Either they name the illness after the person who first described it, for example Bright's disease, or they take a Latin or a Greek root and create an English version. The former, eponym, method is a useful way to have someone remembered by medical posterity. The latter is generally regarded as more scientific or specific. The term 'geriatrics', derived from the Greek words for old age and physician, was coined by an American physician at the beginning of the First World War. Whether or not its originator, Dr Ignatz Nascher, so intended, this elegant label came to denote medical work among elderly chronic sick and incurably disabled people.

No other medical branch or discipline ever started off with a 'brand label' that as it were asked doctors and the public to equate it with the gloomiest outlook. The chronic sick 'image' was clearly reflected in the drab conditions, decaying surroundings and inadequate staffing of the 'old people's wards' in both the old Poor Law institutions and the annexes of the voluntary hospitals. When I set foot for the first time in a typical old people's ward in a large, long-established Lancashire hospital, I felt that I had moved from the twentieth century back to an era when medicine was still in the hands of the alchemists and barber surgeons and the sick were mixed with the poor and the derelict in ancient hospices.

As I recall, the main ward was reached through a heavy fake-panelled door with peeling green paint, on which no ward name or number was visible. Inside, the walls were grubby unplastered brick, thinly disguised with green distemper. High black iron beds jammed close together were parted only by pathetic old wooden or metal lockers. Cotsides on most of the iron beds belied the adult faces of the patients occupying them. Bed coverlets were few and muddy grey in colour. Stone floors, dog-collared naked light bulbs and barred windows completed the picture. Most of the patients were elderly but a few were young people suffering from progressive diseases like multiple sclerosis and muscular dystrophy. The old ones were suffering from all kinds of medical conditions and were often confused and incontinent. The diagnoses on the patient's case sheet were most frequently headed by the term 'senile dementia', irrespective of whether the patient's age was 50 or 90. The nineteenth-century exterior of this hospital building was a fitting match for the interior I have just described.

A few doctors, now regarded as the pioneers of modern geriatrics, realized that three things were necessary if the growing problem of diseases in the elderly was to be met with a dynamic approach. As always, the first need was to inject money into the hospitals so that they could either build new suitably designed wards for the elderly sick or, as in fact happened at first, convert and upgrade the interior of the established wards. The second need was to create a new medical specialty with its own highly trained consultants in diseases of the elderly, in charge of specified geriatric units. These would channel off geriatric problems from the wards and beds of the general medical physicians. The third need was to staff old people's wards with well-trained sisters and staff nurses and not rely merely on the unskilled orderly or nursing auxiliary.

At the Cowley Road Hospital, Oxford, at the West Middle-

sex Hospital, Isleworth, at St John's Hospital, Battersea, and
at Foresthall Hospital, Glasgow, Drs L. Z. Cosin, (the late)
Marjorie Warren, Trevor Howell and (now Professor) W. F.
Anderson began the attack on the chronic sick 'image', and
the destruction of the static and hopeless attitude that tender,
loving care was the only therapy for a sick old person. Their
progress was slow and uphill, so entrenched was the chronic
sick idea. There was heavy opposition from hospital colleagues in the ordinary medical wards, who could not see
the value of spending time, money, energy and bed space
on redundant senior members of the community. They were
loath to admit that the disease pattern in the elderly was
different (see pages 126–30) and might repay special study
(thus repeating the mistake they had made thirty years earlier
with diseases of childhood). Fortunately the progress and
'turnover' of patients in the pioneer geriatric units began to
speak for themselves and persuaded the administrative
medical leaders at the Ministry of Health and on Regional
Boards, that a dynamic policy was worthwhile.

Monies became available for the internal conversion of the
geriatric wards. With a wave of the financial wand, the concrete floors disappeared under non-slip linoleum tiles. Beds
were lowered to a more reasonable height, aluminized and
fitted with fold-away cot-sides. The latter were used infrequently as the care of the patient became progressively more
active. Bed coverlets became blue and orange. Shaded fluor-
escent lights revealed that the open brickwork had vanished
under plaster and two-toned panels. Fewer beds in each
ward allowed more convenient interspersing with formica-
topped patients' lockers. The bars had gone from the windows and the ward was clearly named to establish a viable
identity. If it was an acute assessment ward, the familiar
accessories of modern therapy such as drip stands, transfusion bottles, emergency vials and dressing trolleys were
also apparent; while if it was a rehabilitation ward, an array

of walking sticks, tripods, walking frames, crutches and even a set of parallel bars could be seen happily scattered throughout.

Much later on, in parallel with the slow hospital building programme of successive British governments, a tortoise-like start was made erecting purpose-built geriatric units to replace the Nightingale type of open ward. Such prototypes as the long-stay unit at Heath Lane Hospital, Birmingham, opened in 1963, and the 'race-track' assessment unit at East Suffolk Hospital, Ipswich, opened in 1965, have set the standard high.

AWAY WITH SENILE DEMENTIA

There is an old-established dictum in clinical medicine that it is not sufficient to treat the symptoms of an illness, without making an effort to discover the root cause, and trying to eliminate it. Nowhere is this more applicable than in diseases of old age, where the commonest presenting symptom of any physical or mental illness is confusion. That is to say, clouding of orderly thought in an elderly person may arise from such simply remedied states as constipation, a full bladder and temporary lack of fluid, or mild fever from infection. More serious but still eminently treatable diseases like anaemia, lung congestion and heart disease can similarly fog the old person's thinking. Badly monitored drugs, particularly sedatives and tranquillizers, may also be culprits. Again, more serious illnesses like strokes and tumours and hormone upsets may first appear in an old person in the guise of a confused mind.

As I have said already, a favourite diagnosis in the old chronic sick wards was senile dementia. This implied that the person had a permanent deterioration in his or her personality and mind function due to a chronic, irreversible ageing process. In fact it was often a cover for the doctor's

16

ignorance, or failure to look for an underlying cause of the mental disturbance shown by his elderly patient. Today, however, the medical specialist in diseases of old age is well aware that an acute confusional episode should always be carefully investigated and not be glibly accepted as due to hardening of the arteries and 'senile' brain softening. The diagnosis of senile dementia rarely appears on the modern geriatric patient's case sheet, not because the condition no longer exists but because it is carefully defined: as a progressive deterioration and ultimate disintegration of the aged personality.

In fact, contrary to the case with general medical patients, it is uncommon for a single diagnosis to explain all the features of illness in a given elderly patient. There are usually at least three and up to six disease processes which have to be taken into account. These several diseases may have a direct connexion with each other: e.g. a catarrhal cold becoming acute bronchitis, going on to pneumonia, leading in turn perhaps to congestive failure of the right side of the heart. Alternatively, there might be cirrhosis of the liver, chronic bronchitis, vitamin deficiency, a stroke affecting the left arm and leg, and eye cataracts, all unconnected. As we will see later, the doctor in geriatrics tries to establish the one or two 'important' diseases, i.e. those which threaten the patient's life and welfare more immediately, and treat these first. The others, less urgent, are tackled at judicious periods later. Some may even be left untreated if they are not disturbing the old person for the moment.

Thus when the specialist in geriatrics takes over the old chronic sick wards, his first important task is to sweep away the misleading senile dementia label and review every single case physically and mentally for accurate classification: the essential preliminary to a possible treatment programme for a future outside the hospital ward. New patients admitted to the geriatric unit benefit from this systematic and incisive clinical approach. The news filters back through discharged and rehabilitated patients into the community served by the unit. In this way, geriatric units lose their previous undesirable reputation as points of no return and unwholesome antechambers of the hereafter. They become accepted as the proper place for the accurate diagnosis, treatment and rehabilitation of the elderly sick, under the best possible medical and nursing care and in the most functional and modern surroundings.

BRITISH GERIATRICS SOCIETY (STRICTLY MEDICAL)

English doctors are naturally conservative in their practice of medicine. New treatments and new approaches to therapy are carefully preconsidered and often introduced at a slow pace. This may irritate non-medical observers who see only the good points in proposed innovations and may ignore the undesirable side-effects. The idea of active, even curative, treatment of the elderly sick was revolutionary in medicine. Not surprisingly, there was resistance to this new approach, by hospital doctors, by family doctors and by those in the Public Health services – for several reasons.

In hospital, the elderly sick had usually occupied beds in the care of a general physician whose focus was his younger, 'remediable' patients who could return to work and active citizenship. Lack of time relegated the over-65s to a less positive approach and less complete diagnoses and assessment. Some consultant physicians were unhappy about this differential in priorities while others were less perturbed on the grounds that little could be done for this age group in any case. A few medical 'politicians' were disturbed that a new specialty might appear which would unbalance their own pattern of public–private practice or else disallow them the use of beds to relieve pressure on their acute wards by transferring cases to the 'chronic sick' wards.

In family practice, doctors were inclined to follow the same priorities. They concentrated on children and adults who could obviously benefit by the newer drug and antibiotic therapies and return to school studies and work. They treated their elderly sick warmly and humanely but often echoed the resignation of relatives – 'I know, doctor, she's had a good run anyway' – and agreed that 'tender, loving care' was all that was left.

In the Public Health sector, medical officers of health concentrated their health visitors and district nurses and the home helps on needy families, problem mothers, pregnant women and ailing children, with a low priority for the elderly population.

Doctors are great individualists generally speaking, but recognize the value of organized groups for the dissemination of new ideas and the spread of new knowledge, and as a stabilizing force for their own drive and medical progress. Partly as such a ginger group and partly as self-expression of the medical profession's growing interest in old age, doctors from the three main branches of medical practice came together in 1947 to found the Medical Society for the Care of the Elderly. This society, whose membership was strictly medical, set itself three main objectives. It set out to improve the standards of medical care for elderly patients in hospital and at home. In parallel, it promoted investigation of the problems of old age, both social and medical, and encouraged the study of ageing in broad biological terms.

In 1959, the society's title was altered to the British Geriatrics Society, in conformity with the international nomenclature which now recognized geriatrics as a proper title for study of diseases of the elderly and their treatment. There are over 400 members at the present time, all fully registered medical practitioners with a whole-time or part-time interest in the elderly sick. At twice-yearly meetings, in London and the provinces, it discusses and correlates and sifts old

19

and new facts and figures on every aspect of its subject.

A Ministry of Health pamphlet entitled 'Notes on Form S.H.3. for 1963', referring to the classification of hospitals for the purpose of costing comparisons and financial allocations, defined an acute hospital as having not more than 15 per cent of its beds allocated to the 'excluded departments'. The latter included chronic sick and geriatric. A hospital was classified as chronic where more than 90 per cent of its beds were allocated to the chronic sick. The British Geriatrics Society observed at the time that as long as geriatrics remained an excluded department, its financial resources and facilities and the development of its units would be restricted. Assignment to excluded department status showed failure to recognize that, in an active geriatric unit, the technical nursing load plus the retraining in activities of daily living calls for a high patient–skilled nurse ratio. In addition, the usual drugs, dressings, instruments and special rehabilitation equipment raise the financial needs of the geriatric unit level with, or even above, that of an acute general medical ward.

The Society also recommended the permanent elimination of the unfortunate term 'chronic sick'. It suggested that the group whose progress halted or who required apparently indefinite care should be designated 'long-stay sick (geriatric)' – a rational semantic move in keeping with the newer continuous assessment policy for the aged sick in geriatric units. In 1964, in response to the Society's stated views, the Ministry of Health approached the council of the Society and asked for a suitable definition of geriatrics in Britain today. The Society circulated all of its 400 members, and enthusiastic discussion followed by careful scrutiny of the many suggestions produced a definition. This was approved at an official meeting and read as follows:

Geriatrics is the branch of General Medicine concerned with the clinical and social aspects of acute and long-term illness, the prevention of invalidism and disability, and the care and treatment of appropriate illness in the elderly.

GERIATRIC CARE ASSOCIATION (1963 ALL-COMERS)

The care and treatment of illness in the elderly, as we shall see in subsequent pages, involves many different groups of trained people, not only physicians in geriatrics. It was to some extent inevitable, therefore, that a more broadly-based organization should arise, incorporating the heterogeneous helpers on the pattern of municipal geriatric liaison committees. In February 1962, a number of nurses with a specific interest in geriatrics decided to form a special group. The title for their organization was a reflection of basic thinking – the Geriatric Care Association. Pressure from other interested people resulted in expansion of the membership to include all those professionally concerned with old people, whether in hospital or in the community. While the doctors' own British Geriatrics Society remained exclusively medical, this new Association welcomed to its forum registered and enrolled nurses, welfare and social workers. Hospital administrators, matrons and superintendents of old people's homes also joined the G.C.A. Some doctors were sceptical of the value of such a broadly-based association, viewing it wrongly as a possible rival to the British Geriatrics Society and perhaps diluting the efforts or retarding the progress of the latter. Some remain sceptical but others have rationally changed their views and joined the Association, adding their own enthusiasm and medical knowledge to this cooperative venture.

The first annual conference of the Geriatric Care Association was held in 1963. By the following year's conference, branches had been formed in many towns of the United Kingdom. In 1965, the G.C.A. was publishing its own quarterly supplement on geriatric care, in association with the *British Hospital Journal and Social Service Review*. **This** latter is a well-written informative weekly journal, published through the Standard Catalogue Company, which reaches the widest range of readership in the hospital and administrative and social welfare services. The *British Hospital Journal* supports the aims of the G.C.A., which centre principally on improving the services offered to the elderly. Through its own and sponsored conferences, exhibitions, lectures, and informal talks or study groups, which reach the varied groups under its banner, the G.C.A. educates and stimulates all comers to see 'the other person's problems' and help solve them as far as possible.

In 1966, the Geriatric Care Association, formed with such enthusiasm, felt a draught of opposition to its continued existence and was forced to an agonizing self-reappraisal. Fortunately, the maturity and vitality of its officers kept this diversely crewed ship afloat and steadied its course. The future path and policy of the G.C.A. are still directed to securing a better present and future for Britain's old people.

A WORKING DEFINITION OF GERIATRICS

Everyone has his own definition of old age. Some people think it coincides with retirement and the commencement of the old-age pension, i.e. 65 for men and 60 for women. Some think in a homespun philosophic fashion that you are just as old as you look and as young as you feel. This equates ageing with appearances, e.g. baldness, stooping, wrinkled skin and rheumy eyes. Others, taking a more rigorous line, point out that, biologically, ageing commences from the moment of birth; and (concurring here with the folk-wisdom), that the process may be nearly as advanced in some 50-year-olds as in other 80-year-olds. Attitude is also apt to vary with the age of the observer. Thus to a 16-year-old 35 seems an advanced age, while the same person at 35 takes 60 as the old-age point.

The community's attitude to ageing influences whether a person will admit to others that he or she is old. In primitive tribes, where safety and security depend on young, active leadership, old members may be pushed aside, especially if the tribe is nomadic. Once the same tribe settles down as an agricultural community, the rejected old are likely to become the respected elders. Similarly in civilized states, if the young people set the pace politically and economically, old people are apt to be ignored or pushed into the background. In such conditions admitting one was old could be socially detrimental.

For the hospital, if it is hard to define old age in general terms, it must be harder to define geriatrics in terms of diseases of old age. Some people have tried to reach a definition of old age by comparing average ages in a geriatric ward with those in a general medical ward. In a given hospital community, in the general medical wards 66 per cent of the over-65s were under 75, whereas in the geriatric wards 66 per cent of patients over 65 were 75 or over. The implication would be that true old age does not commence until 75. This fits in with a medical view of ageing holding that old age begins when the complete independence of the adult begins to be eroded. Most geriatricians agree that at the present time, after the age of 80 everyone is partially dependent on someone or some group for continuing the activities of daily living.

Geriatrics has been approached by some doctors on the basis of the common types of medical problem which present in an older age group. In one study the common symptoms for which patients were found to be referred to a geriatric unit included falling about, wetting the bed, mental confusion, weakness of one side of the body and retiring to bed indefinitely with no very obvious diagnosis. The implication of these symptoms might seem to be that all the elderly patients were suffering from hardening of the arteries causing brain softening. In fact, admission of their patients to geriatric units might result in such 'regular' medical diagnoses as (respectively) pernicious anaemia, stone in the bladder, pneumonia, high blood-pressure and an undiagnosed tumour of the bowel.

Another way of looking at geriatrics is to consider the influence of social factors on illness and disability in the older age group. An illness like acute bronchitis, usually treated at home by the family doctor, becomes a case for admission to hospital if the old person has no one living with him or her and no near relatives to help in home nursing. A patient who has had a disability for many years, such as for instance severe arthritis of arms and legs, may depend on the regular efforts of a good spouse or sister for home care. If the latter then in turn becomes ill, this may precipitate the need for the arthritic's admission to hospital. Even such non-crises as moving house or going on holiday may decide the relatives looking after the patient to ask for temporary hospitalization.

Though it may seem like talking in a circle, geriatrics can be defined as the practice of medicine in geriatric units by the geriatric physician and his staff. The important factor here is not so much the age of the patient, as the method of diagnosis and treatment. The method requires, first, that a patient shall be considered as an important individual with a community identity, not just an 'old dear' or 'pop' or 'gran'. Secondly, it calls for as accurate a diagnosis as possible with treatment if treatable. Thirdly, it aims at restoring the patient to the upright position if possible, to a mobile life, if sustainable, and full, integral function in the activities of daily living. All this may sound good, straightforward common sense until you come to try and apply the method to a frail, muddled 82-year-old spinster, living alone in an upstairs flat with an open fire, who breaks her leg, becomes confused and incontinent, is admitted to a geriatric unit for X-ray and assessment and finds warmth, kindness, good

24

food and companionship in an unexpected 'ill wind'. Moreover, the method may clash with the old patient's family's wants – a long-suffering daughter preferring her mother to remain bed-fast and hospitalized so that she can go out to work and lead an independent life; or the wife who prefers her husband to remain chair-fast and unsteady so that she can avoid her marital responsibilities and only has to visit him in hospital for appearances' sake. Fortunately most families have a sense of devotion and a good measure of affection for their senior members, and readily accept their restoration to full function and a return to home life.

A working definition of geriatrics has to be based on full understanding of the multiple medico-social problems of the oldest section of the community, and application of the method which solves these problems. The aim is a return to maximal health and everyday function.

2

WHO ARE THE GERIATRICIANS?

THE GENERAL MEDICAL PHYSICIAN

THERE are three great branches of medicine, popularly called general medicine, general surgery, and midwifery (with gynaecology). In hospital consultant practice, the specialists in these branches are called respectively physicians, surgeons and obstetricians. Under the care of the physician come adult patients (from the age of 14 upwards) suffering from a variety of illnesses which are diagnosed by the physician and treated with rest, diet, drugs and nursing care. If an organ or tissue requires to be cut out, altered or transposed, then the patient will be passed on to the surgeon.

From this, we can see that the care of the elderly sick was previously the responsibility of the general medical physician. The usual arrangement in most general hospitals was that each physician had a set number of acute wards allocated to him for all his medical patients, and a smaller percentage of so-called chronic sick beds, to which he could transfer (young and) old incurable or permanently disabled patients. Such a system was reasonably efficient as long as the numbers of these supposedly 'irremediable' patients remained low and the specialist physician took an active interest in his non-acute patients. Unfortunately the rapid expansion of the Health Service after 1948, and the increasing work load, often prevented such an active interest and promoted *laissez-faire* attitudes in medical and nursing staff on 'non-acute' wards. Add to this the sharp rise in the elderly section of the sick population, with its special medico-social problems, and the need for separate geriatric departments became pressing.

The first generation of geriatricians were all general medical physicians who took a pioneering interest in the special needs of the elderly in hospital. I have already explained how they fostered this interest among their colleagues, through the British Geriatrics Society and among the Regional Hospital Boards, who created separate geriatric units. This produced the second generation of geriatricians, who held primary appointments as consultants solely in diseases of old age. It was this group, themselves trained in the science and art of traditional adult medicine, who discovered and elaborated the different techniques, adjusted therapies, and pinpointed the need for social assessment and rehabilitation of function in the aged sick.

Today's geriatricians – the third generation, as it were – are still trained in the hospitals in the traditional path of general medicine up to the grade of medical registrar. Then, they usually transfer into a geriatric unit to become geriatrics registrars, then senior registrars, and finally consultants in geriatrics, in charge of geriatric units.

A few consultants still hold appointments on a sessional basis, split between general medicine and geriatrics, but this is a diminishing group which will eventually disappear.

PHYSICIAN IN CHARGE OF THE GERIATRIC UNIT

Well-qualified doctor, clear-thinking coordinator, ever ready adviser, untiring enthusiast for making old people better in the shortest possible time: the third-generation type consultant geriatrician must be all these.

The physician in charge of a geriatric unit must be a well-qualified doctor with a higher qualification – e.g. membership of the Royal College of Physicians or a research degree such as M.D. – giving him equal status with his specialist colleagues in hospital. He is not merely the solver of old people's social problems by admitting them to hospital if they have been unattended by relatives, neighbours or friends. In the first instance there must have been an intrinsically medical problem to precipitate the social crisis. The physician in geriatrics must bring his medical knowledge and skill, aided by X-ray and laboratory investigations, to make a diagnosis, and initiate appropriate treatment. On the degree of success here will it subsequently depend whether there is a solution to the social problem.

The essence of geriatrics is teamwork, and the consultant geriatrician is the team's chief coordinator. In a given geriatric department, the medical part of the team will include a senior medical assistant who acts as deputy for the consultant, a registrar who is training for consultantship in the specialty, and one or more junior hospital doctors who carry out the day-to-day medical clerking and clinical procedures on the wards. The nursing part of the team is no less skilled and includes the sister, staff-nurse and student- or pupil-nurse grades. The ancillaries of the team include the physiotherapist with her special methods of muscle and joint retraining, electrotherapy and rehabilitation skills, the occupational therapist with her valuable techniques in retraining for the activities of daily living; and the medical social worker who combines the traditional sympathy and tact of the almoner with a contemporary practical approach to the social, economic and interpersonal problems of the sick elderly. Other members of the team for whom the geriatric physician is the central pivot are the specialist health visitor in geriatrics who, herself, acts as liaison officer with the public health department from which district nurses and home helps emanate; the unit's personal secretary who, in addition to being a medical shorthand-typist, acts as a link in her office between family doctors and relatives outside hospital and the various team members; and thirdly, the lay leaders of such voluntary groups as the W.R.V.S., Old People's Welfare

Committee, and Rotary Clubs, who help the geriatrician at the community end.

The consultant geriatrician requires to be an ever ready adviser. He may be called out to give specialist medical advice for elderly patients in their own homes who are referred by their family doctors. Alternatively, his professional advice may be sought by elderly people attending the out-patients clinics. Any member of his team can request his opinion or suggestions in the host of problems which ill old people present. Moreover, he must define the immediate and long-term policies of the unit and advise the hospital secretary and his administrative team on the working needs of the geriatric department. In the community and in the teaching departments of medical and nursing training schools, through illustrated talks and lectures, he imparts some of his wisdom and experience and tries to clarify for his audiences the broad canvas of old age in sickness and health. Lastly, the consultant geriatrician may be called upon to organize such varied schemes as clinical trials of new drugs or pieces of equipment, or to design new approaches to contemporary problems, or to undertake fact-finding surveys at a community level.

This does not by any means exhaust the functions or capacities of the specialist in diseases of the elderly. In a specialty full of challenging problems, his day-to-day awareness needs to be acute, his response dynamic. We shall see later on how important this is for sick old people.

ROLE OF THE FAMILY DOCTOR

The importance of the family doctor in relation to elderly patients was well recognized by the Review Body on Doctors' and Dentists' Remuneration in their Seventh Report in 1966. They recommended a standard capitation fee for patients over 65 of 140 per cent of the fee for other patients, because of the greater attention elderly patients need from their doctors.

Not only is the overall number of calls greater, but the individual call is liable to take up more of the doctor's time, owing to the often difficult social factors involved, coupled with the old person's slowness in giving his or her medical history, and in undressing for and cooperating in examination.

Since, as we shall see, the hospital geriatric service is orientated towards maintaining the elderly citizen at home, the largest part of geriatric practice falls to the family doctor. Many family doctors, recognizing their preventive as well as curative role, make a regular monthly visit to their over-60s whether they are called or not. This visit is mutually helpful: the old person sees it partly as a social event, while the doctor can observe general health, fitness to manage, state of nutrition and any changes in the personality pattern.

In order to maintain the sick elderly patient at home as long as possible, the family doctor depends on the Public Health department for aid with district nurses and health visitors and also for home helps. His own visits to the patient are more frequent than if the same illness was present in a younger patient. He may be called upon to act as arbiter among indifferent relatives, overtaxed neighbours and over-burdened friends.

As a result of pressure from any or all of the latter, he may have to call upon the local hospital geriatric service. Here, patient and doctor may be baulked by a shortage of geriatric beds, causing unfortunate delay. The strain on the doctor's clinical resources is then considerable.

The family doctor may observe that his old patient, while not suffering from an illness requiring hospital admission, by reason of physical or mental disablement or infirmity requires accommodation in a local authority welfare home. He can refer the patient to the chief welfare officer, who will then visit and advise accordingly.

The general practitioner is also important in relation to the growth of the geriatric preventive health centres which are being set up by progressive local health authorities in various areas. Only the family doctor can refer elderly patients to these centres, which are the Public Health parallel of hospital outpatients departments. The patients in his practice probably include not only those in the general community but those already living in old people's homes or supervised bungalows. These latter also grow older in their sheltered environment, and the doctor keeps a weather eye open for illness or changes in personality, which he may either treat or ask the hospital geriatric unit to assess. Some old people prefer to retain their own family doctor in their new abode, while others join the panel of visiting doctors 'appointed' to attend the home – both schemes have their own merits and may even be combined.

No geriatric unit can hope to function efficiently and humanely, or expect its discharged patients to make a lastingly successful adjustment to life in the general community again, without a close liaison with the patient's family doctor. He needs to be fully informed of the clinical findings, the diagnoses, the treatment and the old person's capacities and expected degree of independence on discharge from hospital. This information he gets usually in the form of a summary note on discharge and a fuller letter later. He must also know what services – e.g. district nurse or home help – are being provided for his patient and what therapies, if any, are recommended by the hospital specialist. With this information and his own full knowledge of the family situation, he can be and is the stoutest prop to his elderly patient.

Unfortunately, as has happened with many of the newer disciplines of medicine, the present and older generation of doctors has had almost no undergraduate and little post-graduate (hospital) experience of the positive geriatrics approach. Experience, refresher courses, conferences and clinical meetings have helped to fill this gap in knowledge, and the newer generation of doctors will have proper undergraduate training in geriatrics in the university departments which will gradually be set up in the various medical schools on the pattern of the Chair of Geriatrics at the University of Glasgow.

Family doctors recognize that it is unwise, and often too late, if they wait for old people to present themselves with an illness or medico-social problem. The nature of the illness or unsatisfactory home circumstances may prevent the aged person visiting the surgery or even calling the doctor by phone or letter. The doctor who gets round to see all the over-65s in his practice at reasonably short intervals, will soon pick out a multitude of illness and social problems which would not have 'come to him'. In group practices, one of the partners may specialize in just this branch or section of the practice and similarly if the doctors are working from a health centre. Sometimes as we shall see later, this 'searching out' work is delegated to the group's health visitor, who has been seconded from the Public Health department.

Having discovered or been presented with illness or a medico-social problem, the general practitioner may call upon the services of the local hospital's consultant geriatrician to assess the urgency for admission to hospital, or to help in the fuller diagnosis and advise on the management. Very many cases, however, are dealt with solely by the G.P., who calls in the necessary services and prescribes the required drugs or appliances on his own judgement and assessment of the problem. If this were not so, the Public Health departments and the hospital geriatric units would disintegrate under an enormous and insupportable load.

THE M.O.H. (MEDICAL OFFICER OF HEALTH) AND THE PUBLIC HEALTH SERVICES

Since 1909, it has been compulsory for all local authorities to appoint a medical officer of health. Most of these are full-time appointments and the M.O.H. is paid directly according to the size of the population which he serves. His is the responsibility for the overall organization and functioning of the many branches of the Public Health department, a responsibility often more demanding in terms of quality, perspicacity and leadership than his salary would suggest.

The M.O.H. is the community doctor in the largest sense. He is usually the principal school medical officer, medical adviser to the child welfare, mental welfare and ordinary welfare departments, and senior medical counsellor to the local authority's health and welfare committees. Under his aegis, too, come the ambulance services, the district nursing service, the home help service and the health visitors department. He is also at the centre of preventive activity like mass radiography against tuberculosis or anti-venereal disease campaigns or smoke control and – to return to our own theme – of help for the elderly in the community. I have listed all these functions to show how important the work of an M.O.H. is on the broadest level of community care, and how many services he in his unique central role can enlist to aid the elderly citizen at home.

Nevertheless, at the time of writing, the future influence of the M.O.H. in several of the departments mentioned above is in great jeopardy. Far from suggesting an expansion of medical influence in the socio-economic problems of the general population, the recent Scottish White Paper and the Seebohm Committee sitting at present* are pointing to changes in welfare and social service departments which are likely to reduce the role of the M.O.H. In geriatrics, this may prove to be an unfortunate move, as it will decentralize even further the ever widening groups of people who play a part in the community care of old people. At least, with the M.O.H. there is some interdepartmental liaison in the Public Health services. Otherwise, the whole

* *Seebohm Committee Report*, July 1968, Cmnd 3703.

trend is in strange contrast to the pattern in hospital, where the many different departments contribute their efforts as a 'team' revolving round the consultant geriatrician. This avoids duplication of work, instructions which cancel each other out and delay in preventive or treatment therapy.

Most areas have a geriatrics liaison committee including representatives of the geriatric and psychiatric hospital departments and their administrative counterparts, representatives of the local executive councils and medical committees, members of the various welfare departments. The M.O.H. sits on this committee and listens to and advises the various groups represented.

The M.O.H. may also set up a preventive geriatrics clinic in the Public Health department buildings to which family doctors can refer elderly persons for a 'check-up' and for X-ray or blood-screening tests. (This is dealt with more fully in chapter 5.)

In many towns, the M.O.H. in conjunction with the hospitals and family doctors has carried out surveys of mental and physical health and elderly persons' housing to obtain a realistic picture of his own area's geriatric problems. He can then apply this information in his own spheres of influence to the general benefit of the senior citizens. He also acts as adviser to the housing department and can promote the building of hostels, bungalows and centres for the elderly or the adaptation of existing property.

Under Section 47 of the National Assistance Act of 1946, the M.O.H. can apply for the compulsory admission to hospital of an old person who requires nursing care and medical treatment but who refuses voluntary admission. The case may be referred to the M.O.H. by the family doctor or a member of the Public Health department and he then applies to the local magistrate for legal powers. 'Sectioning' a patient in is not often resorted to as the M.O.H.'s visit to the patient's home generally results in a voluntary agreement to go into hospital, under the care of the consultant in geriatrics.

Similarly, under the Mental Health Act of 1959, the local mental welfare officer, acting in liaison with the M.O.H., can apply for compulsory admission to hospital where a mentally ill or mentally disturbed old person refuses to enter as an informal patient. The old person is medically assessed by his own family doctor and a psychiatrist before the application is granted. Arrangements for guardianship in a residential hostel can also be initiated by the mental welfare section.

THE GERIATRIC 'TEAM'

I have already mentioned, in passing, the idea of the geriatric 'team'. The necessity for teamwork, involving regular communication and exchange of up-to-date information between the various departments involved in any one patient's care, was thrust upon geriatric units by the pattern of progressive patient care which emerged in the 1950s. No longer could one individual, however skilled or intelligent, encompass all the medical, social, economic and rehabilitation aspects of care of the sick elderly person in hospital. It was soon clear that the consultant geriatrician must take on the focal role in the team, guiding and being guided, advising and being advised at all stages in the patient's progress.

Patients in teaching hospitals often comment dryly on the retinue which follows the 'great consultant' on his teaching ward round. Four or five medical students, student nurse and sister, the house-physician, the registrar and the senior registrar surround the patient whose illness is to be considered. The patient may feel complimented by such interest or alternatively overawed by numbers. In the geriatric ward round, the entire team may be present – the medical and nursing staff as on the 'teaching' round plus physiotherapist, occupational therapist, medical social worker (formerly almoner), unit secretary, and visiting medical or nursing students. If this seems like a trained army on the march, it does not seem to intimidate the sick old person, who most often welcomes such wide attention.

Each member of the team can play a role. Take, for example, the elderly woman who has had a 'stroke' producing partial paralysis of the left arm and leg. She may have become agitated or anxious. The doctor can then prescribe a sedative, the nurse can give reassurance and attend to hygiene and the prevention of pressure sores, the physiotherapist can give passive and demonstrate active exercise for the limbs, the occupational therapist can show the disabled patient how to put on her clothes and the medical social worker can see to such diverse matters as ensuring the rent is paid and the cat taken care of.

Apart from the formal ward rounds, team communication is kept up by notes, memos, telephone calls and weekly or fortnightly inter-staff meetings. The latter are organized on an informal basis with the 'agenda' of patients and problems brought forward by the team members who can collectively suggest solutions. This is the best way to arrive at the flexible 'solutions' which have to be adopted, since there are often too many uncertain or intractable facts to make cut-and-dried statements about the sick old person's future. The inter-staff meetings also allow the airing of unexpected grievances or difficulties which may arise in the traditional hierarchical patterns of hospital management, so that union-like 'demarcation of work' disputes can be resolved.

The 'team' can extend itself into the community by incorporating a specialist geriatric health visitor, seconded by the local Public Health department, who acts in liaison with both the hospital and the family doctor. She may meet team members in groups or at the staff meetings, and also act as a second 'prop' on the patient's discharge. Apart from the health visitor and the consultant geriatrician, home visits with the patient by the hospital's physiotherapist, medical social worker and occupational therapist may be arranged before actual discharge. These team members can then see the patient in home surroundings and advise on simple adaptations – e.g. bed downstairs, rail on one wall, chair at sink – or can arrange for a neighbour or relatives to see the patient and help as required.

The idea of the geriatric team thus emerges not as a pretty label for bemusing the uninitiated, but as a positive tool to help the ill old person to return to community life as fully as humanly possible for him or her personally.

3

AIMS OF THE GERIATRICIAN
(IN HOSPITAL)

THE ASSESSMENT VISIT AT THE PATIENT'S HOME

UNDER the terms and conditions of service of senior medical staff in hospital, hospital specialists and consultants can visit a patient's home at the request of his family doctor. There are officially two separate types of such a domiciliary visit. In the first type, for which the specialist is paid a fee additional to his fixed salary, the visit is made usually in the company of the family doctor, to advise on the diagnosis and treatment of a patient who, on medical grounds, cannot attend hospital. In the second type, known as an assessment visit – and for which no additional fee is payable – the specialist visits the G.P.'s patient to review the urgency of a proposed admission to hospital, or to continue or supervise treatment started or prescribed in hospital, or at an out-patient clinic.

The idea of regular pre-admission assessment grew slowly in the practice of geriatrics. Most departments created waiting lists in the first instance, based on referrals from family doctors or their own outpatient departments. As these waiting lists became longer, it was soon obvious that some sort of review was necessary. Some units did this by either ringing the family doctor to see if the patient or his situation had changed, or arranging for the waiting-list cases to be brought, whether mobile or on a stretcher, to the 'outdoor' section of the hospital, for further assessment.

Other units decided the only way to review the waiting

list was to visit all the patients on it at home. This proved to be so valuable, that the pattern became established of assessment visiting of all cases referred for admission. To some extent a geriatrics assessment visit parallels the paid type of domiciliary consultation since, in assessing the degree of urgency for admission, the specialist is required to make an accurate medical diagnosis and clinical estimate.

Many workers 'in the field' have shown that accurate placement of the sick old person is critically important in determining the eventual outcome and progress. In geriatrics the choice is usually among three possibilities: continued treatment and convalescence at home; admission for further assessment and treatment in a geriatric unit; admission to a mental hospital psychiatric unit for a similar approach. A fourth alternative for the old person reasonably well medically but in need of care and supervision may be a local authority's old people's home.

The geriatrics specialist visiting his patient at home prior to admission can also assess the social conditions and socio-economic position of his patient. Such simple pointers as a long flight of stairs to an upstairs bedroom, or a long walk down a muddy yard to an outside toilet, will guide the doctor on the rehabilitation of, say, a partially paralysed patient. This is obviously very important in planning the re-placement or resettlement of every old person who has to come into hospital for any length of time.

The home visit, moreover, often allows the specialist to meet the relatives, or friends or neighbours, who support the elderly person there. This is also important if the aim is to return the patient to the home environment, as the geriatrician can generally make the relatives a provisional forecast as to how long the patient will be in hospital, how much physical and mental recovery is likely to take place, and what adaptations or support will be called for on the return home.

The specialist, too, can tell the patient and relatives or

friends how long he or she is likely to have to wait before being admitted to hospital, and, whether the old person is being admitted or not, what helping services like district nurse, laundry incontinence service, and home help are available.

Some geriatricians use a 'working code' whereby the medical urgency is assessed as A, B or C and the social urgency is also assessed as A, B or C, where A means acutely urgent, B means very urgent and C means urgent. Thus M/A:S/A on the waiting list against a patient's name means that he has the highest priority for the next bed available. If there is any delay in admitting any of the patients on the waiting list, for example owing to pressure on the beds in winter months, the specialist will revisit and reassess the patient as soon as possible and rearrange priorities, or make other suggestions for management of the case.

The assessment visiting system is not infallible and, in any case, sometimes the patient's illness is so acute, or the breakdown in the social situation is so disastrous, that admission within the hour or day of request will be sought. In that case, the geriatrician may have to take a considered but 'blind' decision to give immediate help, although resettlement of the patient at a later date may be the harder.

THE ASSESSMENT WARD

The pattern of admission to hospital is familiar to most people either from personal experience or from watching television programmes of a medical nature. The admission of an old sick person to an assessment ward involves the same arrival in ambulance or car, and entrance on a stretcher, in a wheelchair or on foot. Where the old person is fit enough to give such personal details as age, religion, address, family doctor and approachable next of kin, these are noted in the personal case record which is made out for every new admission. If unfit to give such details, the patient passes the task on to the relatives or neighbours who have accompanied or followed him or her to the hospital.

The patient is usually asked or assisted to undress if not already in bed wear, and put to bed pending the initial examination by the house doctor. Where necessary a hygienic wash or bedbath is given, provided the patient is fit for it, at the initial admission. The patient's clothes and personal effects are put in a personal bedside locker and he or she is advised on mealtimes, the procedure for toilet needs, and visiting and other ward activities.

As soon as possible after admission, the house physician comes to see the elderly patient. He may already be in possession of many of the social, medical and personal facts of the patient's illness or problem, through the copy of the specialist's letter, to the patient's family doctor after the home visit, which is attached to the new case record. Still, the well-trained house physician usually takes his own medico-social history to supplement the records. Taking a clinical history from an elderly patient is quite different from the standard pattern taught to medical students for adult patients in general medical wards. The old person may be forgetful or slightly deaf, is slower at delivering answers, tends to wander off the point, may misinterpret a question or be preoccupied with such, at that point irrelevant, factors as bowel habits or the value of a patent medicine. Moreover the house doctor finds he has to put 'leading questions' to the patient to elicit symptoms, a procedure which can lead to an inaccurate history for a suggestible patient.

If the patient is recalcitrant or mentally clouded, the house doctor will have to get the history from the attendant neighbours or relatives or friends. He then makes his physical examination with the assistance of a student nurse or ward sister. Again he may find difficulties, in the patient's slow response, or inability to relax, or muddled understanding of his commands, or refusal to be disturbed. Under the circumstances he makes as full an examination as possible of all the body systems – heart, lungs, etc. – and records his findings in the case notes. He then orders any investigations – X-rays, blood tests, urine tests – that seem relevant and either continues the patient's home treatment or initiates such new therapy as seems urgently called for.

The patient may be nursed in bed or allowed to sit out or walk around depending on his or her condition. Attention to hygiene, pressure areas, excretory functions, taking of medicines, recording of patient's temperature, pulse, respiration and blood-pressure, dressings – all these and many other daily ward procedures are carried out by the ward sister and her nursing staff. They will also comfort, reassure and encourage their elderly charges, who are sometimes upset or bewildered by a change from their familiar environment of home, family and pets to a ward life with a different routine. Such upset is more likely if the patient was already confused before leaving home.

The geriatric assessment ward in most hospitals is still usually an (upgraded) version of the open Nightingale-type ward, where the patients' beds are in a continuous row down each side of the ward. As many as thirty-two beds may be housed in such an open ward, so that privacy is hard to come by. The use of movable screens, or fixed-curtain cubicalization, can produce some visual privacy for medical, nursing or hygiene procedures, but no auditory privacy. It is important that all beds should be visible from a nursing-station observation point, but this can still be achieved with glass-windowed partitioning when cubicled wards are purpose-built. Some of the newer geriatric assessment wards have six-bedded, three-bedded and one-bedded cubicles – the latter for the seriously ill or mentally disturbed patients or those who are dying.

The importance of a day-area for patients who are up is

stressed by most geriatricians – some suggest two day-spaces, one for the socially acceptable and one for those showing disturbance of normal social habits. The day-area should have toilet facilities reasonably near and, in any case, there should be adequate sanitary annexes for the patients in the ratio of two water-closets and one bath and shower for every ten patients. Good ward ventilation on the American air-conditioning system is preferable to the 'open-window draughts: closed-window stifling' pattern of many wards. Other recommendations being adopted are sealed non-slip floors, non-glare reflected wide-beam lighting, a variety of chairs (with arms for support), and either a mixture of high and low beds with collapsible protective sides or all beds adjustable for height.

The day-area may also be the dining area for patients who are up. Suitable supporting equipment like walking frames, tripods and crutches must be available in the assessment ward as well as in the rehabilitation wards because, in fact, rehabilitation begins in the assessment ward as soon as the patient is well enough.

PLANNING THE PATIENT'S PROGRESS

The consultant geriatrician may conduct one or two formal ward rounds with his team every week. He is, of course, continuously available to all his staff and visits the ward between times if there is any dramatic change in one of his patients. At the formal round, he also takes a history and makes his own clinical assessment, comparing it with his house doctor's notes. This benefits both the patient – by two opinions – and the house doctor, who is in training. The 'chief', as the consultant geriatrician is called, has the advantage of his previous pre-admission home visit to the patient and his medico-social findings at the time.

For any given geriatric patient the specialist will arrive at more than one diagnosis. In fact illness in the elderly, as already mentioned, is usually multiple, in contrast to illness in other adults and young people, where most of the clinical features can be explained by one diagnosis. An average of three, and up to six, separate disease processes may be distinguished in the one elderly patient, but some of these may be of less immediate importance in the overall picture or not susceptible to any medical therapy yet available. They are not ignored, however, but noted for future reference.

Obviously an illness such as pneumonia or acute heart failure, which immediately threatens life, will be diagnosed and treated on admission by the house doctor, in liaison with his 'chief'. A less urgent but still potentially lethal disease, such as dropsy or uraemia, will be treated next to or alongside the most urgent. As soon as the patient is out of immediate or short-term danger, the medical part of the team will consider more slowly responsive complaints like iron- or vitamin B12-deficiency, calling for injections or small transfusions. Meanwhile the nursing staff will have been 'turning' the patient regularly in bed to avoid pressure sores on back or base of spine, and padding heels and elbows too. They provide bedpans, if necessary, give small enemas or entube the bladder to keep the excretory functions regular. Wet linen and drawsheets are changed as frequently as the hospital laundry service can cope with an increased workload. Special air-cell mattresses, with alternating filling of the cells by an electric motor, can be used for very immobile patients with a high risk of pressure sores.

As soon as the patient is out of any short-term danger, the consultant urges getting out of bed to sit up in a chair. Many geriatrics chairs have a tray front, which can be kept in position while the patient is still relatively weak and possibly liable to lean forward and fall. The alternative is to sit the patient out in the chair with this turned to face the side of the bed, so that any shift forward is then on to soft bedding.

Early movement out of bed, whether just during bedmaking or for progressively longer periods each day, prevents such complications as pressure sores, lung congestion, clots in the lungs, stiff joints (knees and hips especially) and incontinence of bladder or even bowels. Such complications can set a patient back weeks or even months, and must be weighed against many old patients' reluctance to sit out of bed after a recent illness, especially when they have 'enjoyed' attention rarely experienced since childhood days, or if they prefer a passive role in daily living.

The medical and nursing staff, and other members of the team, are on the lookout for any relapse, which may call for a return to bed and interruption of the present line of treatment. Because of this potential 'up and down' swing in the patient's clinical state, the planning of the patient's progress is done on a short-term basis, usually weekly at first, but still with an eye to the long-term resettlement at home or in a hostel or other accommodation.

I have already hinted that the patient's mental state is particularly important in his or her eventual progress. If the patient is deaf or has poor vision, the provision of a hearing aid and the fitting of appropriate spectacles may be a first step in correcting factors that influence mental outlook. A patient who was confused at home may be even more confused in a strange ward with white-coated people and unfamiliar bedding and food. Confusion is the commonest presenting symptom of any illness or disturbance in an elderly person – from an overfull bladder to pneumonia, or from a mild seizure to a growth in the bowel. It does not necessarily imply a permanent disturbance of the mind, and very often, as the acute illness subsides, the old person recovers his or her mental functions of awareness and reasonable concentration. Sedative or tranquillizer drugs are required in the initial confused state, if the patient is restless or agitated, but they are a two-edged weapon as they may be

45

too soporific and produce a very drowsy, more uncooperative old person.

Apart from confusion, an old person may be apathetic, or depressed by his or her medical condition or social problems, or both, and then a skilled psychiatric opinion may be sought. Sometimes a patient's gloomy attitude and failure to admit improvement which is quite obvious even to non-medical observers are expressions of a lifelong pessimistic personality. Sometimes the elderly patient is experiencing kindness, courtesy, regular food and warmth for the first time in many years, and unconsciously resists progress which would mean removal from such a sheltered and 'caring' environment.

While drugs or injections are continued or reduced for the several illnesses present, the next step is from chair to walking – generally with the support of two nurses or physiotherapy auxiliaries at first, then with just one helper, and then using some form of walking aid such as a pulpit-shaped frame, tripod or crutch. Bed-end exercises against a fitted wooden plank at the base of the bed can be carried out, even by partially paralysed patients, using one hand or two. Twin factors used to encourage the patient in the adventure of walking are the lure of the day-area and the appeal of using a real toilet after weeks or months of bedpan or commode. All the staff are encouraged to let these recovering elderly patients do as much for themselves as possible. There is always a tendency for the naturally kind-hearted nurses or ward auxiliaries to do too much for their old charges and rob them of increasing independence all unwittingly. In addition, if there is a shortage of nursing staff – a problem which besets all hospitals but especially those doing geriatrics – the staff are inclined to help patients dress and wash, and whiz them along in wheelchairs to the dining area.

In the day-area, some form of diversional therapy is encouraged, such as the knitting of 'pieces' or embroidery or miniature weaving, or simple stuffing of dolls or making small coat hangers – any procedure which diverts but also makes the patients concentrate a little and use their upper limbs. This is under the supervision of the team's occupational therapist.

In terms of progress there are four groups of patients: those who despite all modern therapy go steadily downhill and die – a relatively small percentage in a given assessment unit; those who make steady progress but need further rehabilitation over walking, balance, negotiation of stairs, and the activities of daily living – who move on to the rehabilitation ward, assuming the unit has one, or may be given a weekend or a week's trial at home to see if they can manage with help from services and relations and neighbours; those who were already in an old people's home and were admitted to hospital because of a medical illness, treatment of which restores them to their previous clinical state ready to go back to the home; and, fourthly, those who make progress from the desperately ill stage to the moderately ill or ill stage but whose condition thereafter remains static – who may be transferred to long-stay accommodation, with the proviso that if they begin to become more mobile, they will be transferred to the rehabilitation wards. There is a fifth group who are really well enough to go home but who are sent to a seaside or country convalescent home, just to build up a little added strength for their return to the community. Lastly there is the – infrequent – case of the old person who is fit for direct discharge from the assessment ward but whose relatives – spouse, children or siblings – refuse to have him or her back. There is usually a reasonable practical excuse such as illness of the relative, widowhood and the need to work, or overcrowding straining accomodation to its limits. But just because these cases are uncommon, and most families make every effort to accommodate their old people somehow, when they do not it is often worth considering whether there may not be a deeper reason. A mother who has been a voluble martinet or a father who has been a lazy wastrel may be reaping the harvest of their own parenthood.

REHABILITATION – OLD AND NEW APPROACH

The development of geriatric rehabilitation wards as separate entities has been slower than the development of the specialty itself. Doctors and nurses both have argued that any geriatric ward can be used to retrain the patient as part of a progress from the horizontal to the upright position, and from the immobile to the ambulant state. These advocates of the all-pattern treatment on the one ward feel that it gives the indigenous nursing staff a chance to tackle all aspects of geriatric nursing under one roof. They also feel that it encourages those less well to take example and heart from those already up and moving. Lastly they consider that it rules out risk of upsetting the elderly patient by frequent changes of accommodation and staff.

Nevertheless, the opposite arguments also apply. Ill or bedfast patients may be disturbed by exercises or occupational therapy activities of patients being rehabilitated on the same ward. Nursing staff does change fairly frequently, in any case, and ward sisters often feel they can best cope and train their student nurses if patients are predominantly at one stage of progress. The elderly patient will, in any case, have to leave the hospital with its familiar faces and its laid-on amenities to return to community life outside. This being so, the rehabilitation ward is a gentler progression from the assessment ward, than straight back home.

The slow promotion of the separate rehabilitation ward can be understood by noting that only five years ago, the most senior geriatrics hospital in the country, with a total bed complement of almost 600, had only 13 male and 20 female beds in its designated rehabilitation ward. (The ratio of male to female reflects the reality of a predominantly female elderly population.) Another reason for the slow growth of these wards is the shortage of physiotherapists, especially those interested in geriatric work, and the even greater shortage of occupational therapists whose work is so complementary.

By the time the elderly patient reaches the rehabilitation ward (or the rehabilitation section of the admission ward), the resettlement plan should be reasonably clear. The patient will be fully independent or semi-dependent in his own home or in a warden-supervised flat or bungalow; or, the patient will be independent for dressing, washing, the toilet, eating, getting in and out of bed, but otherwise need the care of an old people's home; or, the patient will be wheelchair-bound in his or her own or a relative's or an old people's home; or the patient will be semi-bed-bound or . . . but the individual permutations are seemingly endless. Knowing the basic aims, i.e. how many activities of daily living the old person will need to cope with, the rehabilitation ward team can guide and explain and reteach accordingly. Where there is a shortage of physio- and occupational therapists, group classes can be held – on the ward, or in near-by departments with the nursing staff and auxiliaries following up the therapy at ward level. In some fortunate units with a purpose-built day hospital (see chapter 4), the day hospital houses the physiotherapy and occupational therapy departments, which can then spread their influence and aid over the wider network of inpatients and outpatients.

The modern rehabilitation ward differs visually from the uncluttered neatness and obsessive tidiness of the Victorian or even post-war matron's idea of a medical ward. All forms of walking and mobility aids are to be seen by the patients' beds, by the patients' chairs and in use. The pulpit-shaped walking frame, light enough to lift with one finger but strong enough to take a fourteen-stone man's full weight, is the modern wonder appliance. There are very few old patients indeed who do not master its use within minutes. Single-leg walking sticks, tripods, four-legged walking sticks, elbow crutches, French crutches, special custom-built shoes and boots, splints of plaster of paris or polythene, lightweight calipers, toe-raising springs, wheeled walking frames, left- and right-handed wheelchairs – a massive armamentarium is available for such diverse disabling conditions as rheumatoid and osteo-arthritis, paralysis from strokes, weakness from bed treatment, unsteadiness after falls, weakness after broken hips, wasting illnesses, diseases of the nervous system, and many others.

Elderly amputees who have lost one or even both lower limbs may be taught to use artificial limbs on a rehabilitation ward, and the age of, say, 80 has not proved an insurmountable barrier. The orthopaedic and general surgeons may add their services in such cases.

The ward usually has one or more sets of parallel bars, dummy steps and Balkan frames and slings – equipment which is often duplicated in the physiotherapists' department. Sleeping in the rehabilitation ward is preferably on low beds (low for hospitals, that is) and the patient may have a bedside commode if this is the set-up at his or her own home. The occupational therapist sees the rehabilitation patients on the ward to instruct the disabled on dressing and undressing and advise on the use of gadgets to pull up stockings, or Velcro adhesive to replace buttons, or elastic permanently-tied shoe laces, for example. If she takes the patient to her own department, she can assess capabilities, concentration and initiative in cooking and cleaning up in the 'mini-kitchen'. She can also instruct and assess on other daily living functions, like communicating messages to tradesmen or neighbours and ordering household groceries and the like. She can instruct on the use of gadgets for eating (non-spill cups and straws, food-guards on plates) or picking things up or turning things over. She can also provide remedial and diversional activities such as the knitting, basket-work, doll-stuffing, and coathanger-making already mentioned, as well as encouraging the more masculine skills of carpentry and metal work.

The consultant geriatrician and his deputies visit the rehabilitation ward weekly and decide, in consultation with the team, who is ready for discharge and what kind of accommodation is advisable. The patient may be ready for home, in which case the relatives or other attendants are notified as early as possible before actual discharge. Where services like district nurse or home help are considered necessary, the appropriate Public Health department is forewarned so it can arrange visits accordingly. Voluntary services like meals-on-wheels may be enlisted and, where there is a day hospital, weekly attendances there after discharge may be requested. The patient who requires gadgets or a walking aid such as a frame can either purchase these independently or obtain them on loan from the welfare department. A preliminary home visit with the patient accompanied by the occupational therapist, physiotherapist and medical social worker allows these members of the team to see the recovered patient in the home environment and suggest any alterations – e.g. bed downstairs, safety gas taps, ramps to replace steps – that may benefit the patient in day-to-day functions.

If the specialist thinks that the patient is a candidate for an old people's home, he refers the case to the chief welfare officer of the local authority that owns and administers the homes. He or she will visit the patient in the ward and notify the consultant if he thinks the patient is fit and suitable (under the regulations of Part 3 of the National Assistance Act) for one of the homes. He will then 'list' the patient accordingly. Unfortunately, though, the latter may now have to wait three to six months or even longer for actual admission to an old people's home, because of the shortage of such homes in most areas. The consultant geriatrician will then have to decide with the patient and relatives, whether the patient can still be discharged to his or her own or relatives' homes temporarily. With goodwill and full support from services and day hospital (where there is one), this can often be managed at least for a short time. This prevents such patients 'blocking' the geriatric beds and delaying the admission of ill patients from the community. On reflection, there seems little doubt that local authorities, who depend on the ratepayers for their monies, have failed to keep pace with the transformation of geriatric units and their higher 'turnover' and well-discharge rates. I will not point the obvious moral.

After six or nine months of rehabilitation, it becomes obvious in a percentage of the patients, that they are going to remain too mentally dull, confused or disorientated, or alternatively too heavily physically disabled by their illness, to lead even a semi-independent existence outside a hospital-type environment. Such patients will be considered for, and eventually transferred to, long-stay ward accommodation. Alternatively, if a patient is financially very well off, he or she (or the relatives) may opt for care in a nursing home or eventide home. Sometimes, to the respectful amazement of the geriatric team, relatives will take home and care for and nurse a very disabled patient – a tribute of affection and love that transcends the call of duty.

LONG-STAY CARE – SOME NEW IDEAS

I have previously pointed out that patients admitted to geriatric units usually come in from their own or relatives' homes or old people's homes. As yet I have not drawn attention to the fact that patients are also referred for geriatric care from other units – general medical, surgical, orthopaedic and gynaecological – in the serving hospitals, and that it is the consultant geriatrician's job to visit, assess and place these referred patients, too. I have chosen this point to mention the fact because so often the reasons for referral are that the other unit's specialist feels that he can do no more for the patient, that he or she is not amenable to therapy in his own unit, or will require to stay in hospital for terminal care (in the case of cancer patients) or (in the case of the disabled or confused) an indefinite long period. These referrals are very often, that is, of the 'chronic sick' type, suggesting that the 'chronic sick–geriatric' equation – discussed in the first chapter – still lingers in the minds of hospital colleagues.

The long-stay wards are the direct successors of the chronic sick wards in that they house and nurse patients who do not make progress in the assessment–rehabilitation programme already outlined. Because of ineradicable mental or physical disability, or failure to respond to treatment, such patients require indefinite nursing with intermittent medical attention and cannot be discharged to their own or an old people's home. The long-stay wards in many geriatric units are housed in either the least desirable – from an active therapeutic and functional viewpoint – of hospital property such as eighteenth- or nineteenth-century converted Poor Law institutions; or now defunct fevers or tuberculosis wards in out-lying hospitals, which are too substantial to pull down but too remote for any but long-stay geriatric cases.

Nevertheless Regional Boards have spent some monies on these long-stay wards, on decoration of walls, better ventilation, better lighting, improved sanitary facilities with disposable bedpans and bottles, proper locker accommodation, curtains, carpeting of day-areas, cantilever bedtables. 'Open visiting' facilities are provided. On other wards with more acute nursing, or busy rehabilitation programmes, a 'long visiting day' is less welcome, at least to the staff. On long-stay wards, however, visitors are very welcome to fill up the long hours and help patients in simple tasks. Voluntary bodies like the W.R.V.S. or Women's Institutes often help to provide pictures and wall decorations, or a mobile sweet or clothes shop, or entertainments like choirs or glee-groups. Filmshows are given, and mobile library facilities are available for those who can still read with enjoyment. The nursing staff take such suitable occasions as Christmas, Easter, anniversaries or patients' birthdays to organize a 'party' and a special tea.

No nurse or doctor will deny that nursing their patients on a long-stay ward calls for the three Vs: vim, vigour and vitality. A high incidence of incontinence, overweight or severely crippled patients to be carefully handled, a percentage of confused or garrulous patients to be cajoled and calmed – all this calls for nurses combining to an exceptional degree full knowledge and application of basic nursing skills with their traditional courtesy, kindness and sense of duty. The state-enrolled and senior state-enrolled nurses along with nursing auxiliaries, are the backbone of the staff who cope with this 'irremediable' group of patients. Doctors visit as required to treat any specific medical illnesses, and the consultant or his deputy will visit regularly to see that the patients are not deteriorating medically, and whether in fact some might not profit now from a second try at rehabilitation. He may also do a 'teaching round' for the pupil nurses, who can then better understand diagnoses and their patients' prospects, or lack of them as the case may be.

The actual numbers of long-stay patients appear to be increasing, which is not surprising considering the much increased 'turnover' of patients in geriatric wards in the last decade. One geriatrician has said that as many as one in five of all elderly admissions require permanent hospital care, but this proportion must vary from place to place. Since many geriatric units already have a total bed complement which is less than the recommended minimum figure per 1000 population, they do not wish to increase their numbers of long-stay beds to the detriment of assessment and rehabilitation beds. As a 'solution' to this problem, some years ago several geriatricians suggested that long-stay wards might be taken out of the present context of geriatric units and administered as separate 'hostels or homes for the elderly sick' paralleling National Health Service patterns for convalescent homes. The problem of providing nursing staff would still arise.

Despite such splinter-group suggestions, it looks as if long-stay accommodation will remain part of the geriatric set-up for some time yet. In 1963, Birmingham Regional Hospital Board gave a lead with the opening of the first prototype purpose-built long-stay unit in an L-shaped design, allowing both sexes to be accommodated in the one unit when only one is required, with sixteen beds in each wing of the 'L'.

Apart from long-stay nursing, the general question of nursing staff in geriatric units has been a difficult one for many areas and hospitals. Because of the basic nursing involved in acute and long-stay cases, because of the fact that even when other units' wards are 'quieter' (holidays and Christmas) geriatric wards are full, because of the cases of incontinence and mental disturbance met with in all geriatric units, and because of the relative absence of the 'dramatic' element, geriatric nursing has previously been regarded as heavy-going, unrewarding, unpleasant, uninteresting and unimportant. This attitude has been common from high to low places and resulted in the iniquitous 'oh, just another pair of hands will do' attitude of matrons and sisters in the not-so-very-distant past.

Fortunately, nurses have been infected by the attitude of the geriatricians and impressed by the effectiveness of better diagnosis, more careful assessment and controlled drug treatment. In many places, rehabilitation methods have been accepted as of nursing interest and part of a nurse's duties on geriatric wards. Aids with the 'heavier' part of the work, such as mechanical lifting gadgets and hoists, and others to ease the unpleasantness of incontinence – plastic sheets, absorbent disposable pads, disposable bedpans and bottles – have been introduced. Proper teaching ward rounds for student and pupil nurses, with formal lectures on geriatrics, give nurses in training an all-round picture of the aims of the new specialty we are outlining in these chapters.

Previously, untrained orderlies and nursing auxiliaries were thought to be satisfactory basic staff for geriatric wards. Their help and kindness and hard-working approach was and is much appreciated, but the new forms of care and treatment call for a larger patient–skilled nurse ratio. The effect of the Platt and Salmon reports*, and their effectiveness in improving recruitment to nursing as a whole, remains to be seen. In geriatrics, the importance of influencing the bodies that control nursing training to allow longer periods of training on geriatric wards, and the need to restress the challenge and rewards of nursing the elderly sick back to health and mobility for a return to the community, are well recognized by those already converted to the cause. Whether creating a new special certificate of geriatric nursing in addition to the standard diplomas, would help, is worth considering in any future nursing career survey.

From what I have been saying, it will be clear that selection of nurses who could make a career in geriatrics can never be easy. There is said, too, to be a traditional antipathy of the young towards the elderly after the dissolution of the child–grandparent bond that tends to appear at puberty. Nevertheless I am impressed by the kindness and understanding shown by many student nurses towards their elderly patients. In particular, the cheerful encouraging extroverted nurse in a rehabilitation unit can often help mobilize the apathetic or depressed old man or woman who

* *Platt Committee Report* on Reform of Nursing Organization and Education, 1964; *Salmon Committee Report* on Management Structure in Nursing, 1966.

does not respond to the advice and treatment of the medical attendants. As in other walks of life, education, and understanding of the illness and its effects on the individual patient's feelings and outlook, will increase the numbers of those who can satisfactorily nurse the elderly.

Care of long-stay patients, and those with anti-social or relatively unwholesome tendencies, calls for nurses older in experience, and emotionally more mature and stable, than nurses in adolescence.

4

AIMS OF THE GERIATRICIAN
(IN THE COMMUNITY)

KEEPING THE PATIENT AT HOME

IN the earlier days of the National Health Service, the general
orientation was hospital-based, so that the fastest expansion
in manpower and equipment took place in hospitals –
although actual new hospital building was extremely slow –
and outpatient and inpatient hospital waiting lists grew
enormously. Casualty departments found themselves doing
minor surgery and emergency work previously the province
of the family doctor. Mothers were encouraged to have their
babies in hospital rather than at home. In the last few years,
however, the orientation has shifted back to the family
doctor service and treatment at home wherever possible.

Where children and non-elderly adults are concerned,
most minor illnesses like fevers, bowel upsets, colds, 'flu
and urinary infections, and several major illnesses like
rheumatism, pleurisy and mild heart disease, can be treated
at home – since there is usually a healthy parent or spouse to
act as a temporary nurse and medicine-giver. In the case of
elderly people at home, even a minor illness like 'flu or a
bowel upset may produce a major social problem in care and
management. Active help to supply meals, fluids, nursing,
laundry and prescribed medicine is very often unavailable
because the old person lives alone (widowed or unmarried);
or the spouse is old and frail and in need of support; or the
old person is living with even older brothers or sisters; or
the old person is dependent on equally aged neighbours; or

the old person has a bedroom upstairs with the toilet downstairs or in the backyard; or the old person lives with a spinster daughter or bachelor son who has to go out to work to support the household; or . . . but again there are many permutations of the basic problem: lack of readily available help.

Keeping the elderly patient at home through even minor illness or upset puts a strain on those normally helping the old person when well, and calls for the family doctor to supply more than a slip of white paper with the appropriate antibiotic prescription on it. He will have to enlist both voluntary and local authority help – but old people, just like any other group, prefer to remain in their own familiar surroundings with their own familiar faces, objects and pets, if at all possible.

Let us take a random example of an old lady, widowed, in her late 70s, living in a two up–two down terraced house with steep stairs and an outside toilet, with elderly neighbours on each side and with a married daughter eight miles away. She has a dizzy spell one morning and finds that she has slight weakness of her left arm and left leg, and lies down on the sofa in the front room. We can picture subsequent events and the possible voluntary and local authority help that will be invoked. The neighbour who normally pops in each morning notices that Mrs A has not taken in her milk. She goes in and finds her friend on the sofa, and hears about the dizzy spell and the weak left side. She makes Mrs A comfortable with a pillow and a handy overcoat in lieu of bedcovers and gives her a cup of tea and some bread and butter. She then leaves her and contacts another neighbour, who sends her teenage girl to the corner shop to ask the grocer to phone Mrs A's family doctor. If the married daughter is on the phone she is called too – if not, she will have to be reached by police message or a letter posted.

Dr S comes after lunch and tells Mrs A she has had a slight

seizure but is recovering nicely. He checks her blood pressure and gives her a prescription for tablets or a syrup. He asks her and the neighbour what help is available. The neighbour explains that she herself has arthritis and sugar diabetes and can't really nurse Mrs A. She points out that Mrs A has not been able to 'hold her water' and there are no proper laundry facilities; also the toilet is outside and the bed upstairs. Equally, the married daughter lives eight miles away and has three children herself so Mrs A could not be taken there to convalesce.

The family doctor says he will contact the local authority about help, and Mrs A mentions she does not like the idea of being alone at night, having just had a slight stroke. She asks if she has to stay in bed for a long time and he tells her that she should be sitting out a little in two days' time and starting to walk a little after that. He leaves Mrs A, makes a visit to another patient, then calls in at the Public Health department where he speaks to several different 'helping agencies'. He speaks to the district nursing supervisor, who promises to send a district nurse later in the afternoon to attend to Mrs A's hygiene and pressure areas and check her pulse and temperature. On her way, she will pick up some absorbent inconti-pads to save the linen while Mrs A is wetting herself. She may also bring a bedpan with her. The district nurse will then go in daily or as often as appears necessary.

The doctor speaks to the home helps supervisor, who promises that she or her deputy will visit and assess how much home help is needed. He speaks to the area health visitor or specialist geriatrics health visitor (if there is one available), who promises to visit and give her expert advice. She suggests that Mrs A might like her bed brought downstairs to replace the uncomfortable sofa, and perhaps she can arrange for the Red Cross to provide a bedside commode for the next phase when the patient is sitting out. Dr S mentions that

Mrs A is a bit afraid of being alone tonight, so the health visitor says she will contact the local old people's welfare committee to see if they can provide a night sitter for tonight. She also asks if he has spoken to the district nurse about the laundry service for incontinents – but in any case she will see to it for him.

He then goes to the welfare department and tells them that it looks as if Mrs A is going to be a candidate for an old people's home when she recovers. One of the welfare officers agrees to visit her and also asks the doctor if, in the meantime, she needs any aids to getting about like a walking frame or crutch or tripod.

The doctor says he thinks she may need a crutch or tripod but he will let them know after the physiotherapist from the county mobile physiotherapy service has visited in a day or two with a view to getting Mrs A on her feet again. Lastly he contacts the W.R.V.S. about providing meals-on-wheels two days a week to dovetail with the home help cooking a couple of other days. He hopes that Mrs A's daughter will also manage to visit occasionally to furnish meals.

This typical example shows the wide cross-section of local authority and voluntary agencies who are available and keen to help the family doctor treat his old patient at home. If the situation breaks down medically or socially, however, the hospital's consultant geriatrician will be asked to visit and assess for admission to hospital or a home.

HOME SERVICES – THE DISTRICT NURSE, THE HOME HELP, ETC.

The district nurse, or home nurse as she is sometimes called, is a familiar figure in most rural and urban communities and has been so, from the days when she walked to her patients or rode on her bicycle. Today she is more likely to have her small car or mini-van. She works under the direction of the superintendent of the district nursing service, part of the Public Health department, and is available to visit the sick of all ages at the request of a patient's family doctor.

At one time, the district nurses were all state registered nurses but now this important front-line task force has been increased and widened by the addition of state enrolled nurses. It is sometimes overlooked that men, too, can become home nurses and the male district nurse is especially useful in geriatrics work, where male patients sometimes refuse the help of females in personal hygiene.

Of all visits to sick people that district nurses make, up to 70 per cent are to people in the over-65 age group. This means that the district nurse is the family doctor's 'right-hand man', whose many duties include giving injections (antibiotics, insulin, etc.); dressing ulcers on heels, legs, and back, for example; administering enemas in cases of severe constipation; bed-bathing the weak or incontinent; helping frail patients into a bath; replacing inconti-pads; checking on skin pressure areas; preventing pressure sores as far as possible, and . . . a myriad unwritten helpful measures that are undertaken often in cramped, ill-lit, ill-ventilated surroundings, with the overweight as with the lean. Moreover she almost invariably becomes a trusted friend, who is relied upon to listen to other problems and advise on family situations not always within the scope of her training and mandate. She is ready to advise the old patient's attendants on simpler nursing and dietetic measures, and her sympathy, kindness and active help can turn the tide for her elderly charge.

She can also recommend to the local authority patients who might benefit from a convalescent holiday. Her visits can be as frequent as twice daily but may be restricted by a general shortage of district nurses or the pressures of, say, a winter 'flu epidemic. Sometimes her visits are restricted to one-item attention – e.g. giving fortnightly injections of vitamin B12 in pernicious anaemia; but even then, the good district nurse will observe any need for general nursing care and report it to the supervisor and family doctor.

The home help service is part of the health and welfare services of the local authority, but is purely a permitted service. That is to say that the local authority has powers to provide such a service but is not compelled to do so. In fact, most local authorities do run a home help service. It is organized by the home help supervisor, who receives requests from all branches of the Public Health department and the family doctor service, to provide domestic help in households where illness or medico-social problems make it necessary.

Once a request for help has been received, the supervisor or her deputy will visit and assess the situation for herself. She will decide how many hours a day and how many days a week (the service may not be available at weekends or Christmas or other bank holidays) her home help will attend the household. When the service first started, assistance for old sick people formed, in most areas, a relatively small part of the home help work. Today it forms the larger part. The number of home helps employed by the service varies according to the economics of the Public Health department (which depends on ratepayers' money), the general availability of womanpower, and economic conditions in the community, such as the counter-attractions of short hours for larger pay in industry.

The home help may attend for say, one hour five days a week, or one half-day a week, or . . . whatever permutation the home help supervisor thinks is best. There is sometimes a conflict between the requests of family doctors, geriatricians, and nurses, who feel that more home help is needed if an old person is not to get worse, and the actual time recommended by supervisors who feel they can only provide a service to meet the problem at the present point. This prophylactic-versus-therapeutic dilemma for home help services might be resolved by better liaison among the various groups, and by giving a medically-slanted training to home help supervisors.

Male home helps have also been recruited in some areas, and proved their worth. The main duties of all home helps include shopping for the disabled or ill old patient, cleaning, washing (within certain limits) and cooking. The service is chargeable for according to the income of the household, but an old person who is already receiving supplementary pension from the Benefits Commission of the Ministry of Social Security can recover the costs.

Some authorities are trying to extend the service to weekends and bank holidays, when neighbours and relatives go on holiday and the old patient needs the services even more. They can also provide a temporary night-sitter service in some cases, to complement the voluntary group's sitters already mentioned.

There are several other home services which I shall discuss in ensuing chapters, all aimed at keeping the old person – sick, disabled or just frail – happily at home.

HEALTH VISITING IN GERIATRICS

A health visitor is a highly qualified trained nurse (usually holding the State Registered Nurse and State Certified Midwife diplomas) who has taken a year's course in social medicine leading to the granting of a health visitor's certificate. The department of health visitors usually has a superintendent and is part of the staff of the medical officer of health in the local authority. With her nursing background and social medicine training, the health visitor is the ideal person to carry all aspects of preventive medicine and nursing into the community. The health visitors are given designated areas to visit, and ascertain and advise on the well-being of selected families, even where there is only one person in the 'family unit'. Their work can be seen as in some ways complementary to that of the district nurses but stressing the preventive side of medical care.

The pattern of health visiting is changing and in many areas the health visitors are seconded to family doctors in group practices, to work with them and help seek out and solve socio-medical problems. They spend a large part of their time with mothers who are not coping or who are having difficulty with their children, or who are still tiros in the mothercraft game. They attend post-natal and child welfare clinics, and follow up children with potential problems due to physical defects. They also attend elderly persons in the community, giving advice and help on normal or diabetic or low-calorie diets, on methods of cooking to retain vitamins, on home safety where steps, lighting, carpets, shelves are possible dangers, and on matters of hygiene pertaining to the skin, the excretory functions, ears and feet. They ensure that the old person has the statutory or supplementary benefits from the state to which he or she is entitled, and advise on which departments can supply various aids.

In some areas the public health department seconds a specialist geriatrics health visitor to the local hospitals' geriatric unit. She sees the elderly patients before discharge and can follow up at home, ensuring that they are carrying out the prescribed therapies and managing a satisfactory existence within the limits of any disabilities and the available home services. She can warn the family doctor if the patient appears to be relapsing and they can liaise with the hospitals' geriatrician.

A distinguished geriatrics health visitor speaking at a nursing conference suggested that health education in geriatrics – for relatives, neighbours and friends-in-attendance and for the elderly person concerned – involved 'unteaching': simply explaining, tactfully, that so many disabilities which were ignored or untreated because 'it's just age', could be corrected or modified. Deafness, poor vision, bad feet and falling hair are obvious examples of these. She suggested that, if it is accepted that old people are fixed in their ways and not likely to be moved by appeals to logic or 'changed times', then middle age, i.e. the pre-retirement phase, is the time to explain and advise, and correct negative attitudes.

Health visitors do, in fact, play a main role in the preventive geriatrics health clinics which are slowly spreading throughout the country (see chapter 5). They also educate and guide by giving talks to pre-retirement groups, over-60s clubs, church guilds, and indeed to any interested group. Their collective value in preventive geriatrics is very high indeed.

THE DAY HOSPITAL

The growth of day hospitals in the Health Service could equally well have been mentioned in the previous chapter or in the chapter which follows, because their work cuts across hospital and community barriers and also has a preventive aspect. The first-ever day hospital in Europe was initiated by the Russians as a psychiatric project as long ago as 1932. Its significance was temporarily lost in the politico-economic problems and the sulphonamide antibiotic wonder-drug medicine of the 1930s and 1940s.

In Great Britain, although outpatient treatment at hospital dispensaries and family doctors' surgeries had been accepted since before the days of the Poor Law, the idea of inpatient treatment on a day basis was slow to be accepted. The first English day hospital was again a psychiatric venture, at a London mental hospital in 1946. In 1952, the Oxford Geriatric Unit, a pioneer of many aspects of medicine for the aged, established the first purely geriatric day hospital. Subsequently the idea spread among geriatric and psychiatric units throughout the British Isles.

As a parallel venture, voluntary groups and local organizations, often with the blessing of local corporation grants, set up day centres and day clubs. These draw their members on the basis of an age group (e.g. old men's clubs or over-60s centres), or of a handicap (e.g. clubs for the deaf or disabled), and members attend for essentially social or socio-economic reasons. Living alone or with relatives at work all day, needing warmth and companionship, desiring active or passive forms of recreation, all are good reasons for attending the day centre or club. The members usually pay a subscription whether the club has a grant or not. They come on foot, by wheelchair, by bus or hired car.

The day hospitals, in contrast, take their patients for medical or medico-social reasons only. The day hospital building itself is usually sited in the hospital grounds near to, or adjoining, or as an integral part of its fostering geriatric unit. The building may be adapted from an existing structure or purpose-built to a specified design. A day hospital is essentially a '9-to-5' (or more realistically 10-to-4) affair. Patients make themselves ready – with or without the aid of relatives or friends – and an ambulance specially chartered by the department (in agreement with the ambulance service) picks up all those in a given area and delivers them to the day hospital. After morning coffee or tea on arrival, the patients participate in an enjoyable pre-arranged programme of activities, treatment, meals and rest phases. The ambulance returns later in the day to take them back to their own homes.

A typical day hospital has a treatment room (for medicines, injections, dressings and physical examination by the doctors); an occupational therapy room – which may also serve the main inpatient geriatric wards – for diversional leisure work, or remedial work for disabled limbs and muscles, or training in daily living activities; a physiotherapy room – also able to serve inpatients – for group and individual games, exercises and rehabilitation work, like walking, going upstairs, lifting objects; a rest room; suitable sanitary annexes with a bath/shower room; a dining hall – separate or doubling as the physiotherapy room; sisters'-cum-medical social workers' soundproof office for interviews and liaison.

Once again, then, the 'team' is at work, with *ad hoc* additions like the chiropodist, the appropriate ministers of religion, hairdresser, and voluntary visitors and helpers. Patients are referred to the day hospital from the hospital's own unit for a follow-up period of one, two or three days per week for one to six months after discharge, attendance being reviewed at appropriate intervals by the 'team'. They may also be referred to the geriatrician for possible attendance, through family doctors and health visitors, or from out-patients or Public Health preventive clinics.

As long as the growth of home and hospital geriatric services is restricted by lack of finance, beds, staff, etc., the day hospital will flourish as a project which lets patients enjoy the benefits of in-hospital treatment while remaining part of the community.

In case I have given the impression that geriatric patients either in hospital or attending the day hospital never breathe fresh air or enjoy daylight and sunshine, I should explain that when the weather is appropriate, outdoor activities replace indoor rehabilitation work. Some day hospitals and many ordinary hospitals have pleasant lawns and paths which can be used for this purpose or for the 'rest periods'. Unfortunately appropriate weather for old people's outdoor activities is limited in the British Isles but the use of glass-fronted sun lounges with maintained warmth can simulate the outdoor situation.

The aim of a day hospital is to follow up rehabilitation initiated in hospital or in the outpatient department; to sustain patients likely to relapse or needing extra support to keep going; to give temporary relief to relatives of mildly disturbed old people; and to observe the effects of drug treatment for the hospital medical department. There are no really typical complaints for which patients are pre-eminently referred to the day hospital; such varied conditions as slight strokes, arthritis, anaemia, mild heart complaints, nervous diseases and mild confusion may be represented.

SPECIAL ACCOMMODATION FOR THE ELDERLY COMMUNITY

A number of critical surveys in different parts of the United Kingdom have shown that not only is the standard of housing accommodation unsatisfactory for the general population, but the elderly section of the population fare worst of all. The elderly community is basically a fixed-income group whose members do not spontaneously move from low-rent substandard property to better accommodation at much higher rents. Moreover old people dislike a change of environment and the attendant change in neighbours, and in shops, leisure sites, pubs, and familiar transport numbers and times, which they have known for a quarter of a century or more.

A look at housing reveals that the old person who may be slow in limb movements and unsteady on looking up, have poor vision, some imbalance on steps, stiffness of the spine and a poor sense of smell, and who perhaps complains of rheumatic pains in the joints, may be living alone in a very old five-roomed house with high shelves, dimly lit hall and stairs, bedroom and toilet upstairs with steep steps and only one handrail, low sinks and low W.C., a gas cooker that does not light automatically, and poor damp-coursing. Moreover the house may have railless outside steps and be far from shops or public transport. That is just one example of how accommodation can be grossly unsuitable for an old person with a particular combination of disabilities. Other forms of housing – stone cottages, old terraced property, slum tenements – can serve other combinations equally ill.

At one time, if an old person became incapable of managing at home but did not require hospital admission, the only alternative was residential accommodation in an old people's home. Under Part 3 of the National Assistance Act, 1948, the local authority is required to provide such residential accommodation for persons who by reason of age, infirmity or other circumstances are in need of care and attention which is not otherwise available to them. The local authority is also under an obligation to provide temporary accommodation in unforeseen circumstances like fire or collapse of buildings, or to allow relatives of old people to take a short holiday.

Local authorities often prefer the term 'welfare home' as a synonym for old people's home. The welfare home has to cope with a wide range of residents, from those whose health is sufficient for independent housing, as for instance supervised bungalows, to those whose disabilities or infirmity calls for geriatric hospital accommodation. Moreover the welfare homes are also expected to care for residents during minor illnesses or, at the other extreme, when they are not expected to live more than a few weeks: doing what would 'normally' be done for a patient in his or her own home. Unfortunately many welfare homes are short of staff and if, say, there is a brisk minor epidemic of colds or 'flu, such staff as there are cannot undertake the nursing of a quarter of the residents as well as their ordinary duties. So there will be requests to the geriatrician for hospital admission of some of the cases.

Old people who require welfare home accommodation are often referred by their family doctor, health visitor, district nurse, voluntary organization visitors, or ministers of religion, or may simply suggest it themselves to relatives. An officer of the welfare department of the local authority visits and assesses whether the welfare home is the appropriate solution – sometimes 'listing' the old person straight away, sometimes suggesting a period of rehabilitation in a geriatric unit. As I mentioned in chapter 3, there is often a delay in the old person being admitted to a welfare home, because of a shortage of places. Most local authorities are increasing their welfare home building programme within the limits of the economic situation for the ratepayers.

In the original choice of residents for the welfare homes, it was expected that they would be able to walk unaided (or with stick or frame), get in and out of bed unaided, wash and dress and carry out personal hygiene unaided, eat unaided and be able to enjoy full recreational activities. However, we are experiencing a continuing rise in the actual age of elderly people – into the 80s and 90s – seeking welfare home accommodation; and this apart from the ageing of residents already in the homes. The need for a home which could take patients requiring some help in daily living activities, not perfectly continent, needing help to walk – such a need became pressing. Many local authorities have therefore built homes for such 'frail, ambulant' patients/residents, where the staff are nurses or ex-nurses and are supervised by a nursing-trained matron.

Local authorities in many areas have also taken on responsibility for the mildly confused or forgetful old person who does not require continuous nursing or medical therapy. The mental welfare homes they have set up are proving a great help in resettling patients who need not be in hospital geriatric or psychiatric units, but who are too confused to live a normal community life in a welfare home.

Local authority welfare homes are not 'free' but the standard weekly rate to live there can be reduced if the resident's finances are limited. The sum deducted must leave a residuum for any small-scale personal needs. The home itself must provide regular meals; satisfactory one-level accommodation (usually rooms with two beds or more) on the ground floor (unless there is a lift); full recreational facilities such as lounges with radio, TV, books, diversional pursuits, gardens;

and such personal needs as cigarettes or tobacco, sweet-meats, and clothes and footwear. Old people are accommodated in welfare homes in their own area, in their own familiar locale, if at all possible.

Forward-looking authorities have realized that other forms of accommodation, purpose-built or adapted, can be suitable for elderly people. Thus warden-supervised bungalows and flatlets – groups of say, ten or twenty with a resident warden who makes sure that fires are lit, food is taken in, residents are not 'poorly' – are being built. Sometimes these flatlets or bungalows are built adjacent to new welfare homes with a connexion to them by warning bells or Tannoy call system – here the home warden doubles as the bungalow warden. Sometimes houses are converted into bedsitting rooms with a communal dining-room and lounge and a resident warden – a good way of making use of large houses which are still in good repair but too large and too expensive for old people to keep up individually.

A number of voluntary organizations and private-enterprise societies have converted old large houses, or built property, on this pattern, which thrifty old people with some capital can buy on a sort of 'mortgage' basis or else rent at a reasonable rate.

The importance of safety factors like good lighting, good ventilation, non-slip carpeting or flooring, safety gas or electric appliances, suitable heating of all rooms, double-railed stairs, ramps or short steps, raised or railed W.C.s, and many other commonsense measures, is realized by those who are involved in accommodating or resettling old people – but the same measures are equally important in ordinary homes.

There has been some argument as to whether old people's bungalows should be built in their own self-contained little development, or as part of an estate on which younger people are also housed. The trend seems to be towards keeping such housing units within the general community, so that the old people can still enjoy a panorama of children, shops, gardens, perambulators, housewives, and near-by public transport and pubs and cafés, yet live safely and comfortably in purpose-built accommodation.

Private nursing homes for the elderly have been established in most parts of the country, taking patients who can afford the weekly fees, of up to £25 in some cases; but these are often full and have a waiting list as well. Moreover patients there may eventually use up their savings capital, following which requests for admission to the geriatric unit are made.

Short-stay homes, taking single persons or married couples who require, say, a month's break from self-care but cannot afford an expensive (possibly unsuitable) hotel holiday, have been established by the British Red Cross. The fees are very reasonable, but like the welfare homes, these Red Cross ones can usually only cater for the fairly fit, mentally alert, and independent. Many religious bodies finance, build and support their own old age homes for the benefit of the elders of their individual creed.

Lastly, I should mention the boarding out schemes for the elderly. On a sort of reversed foster-parent pattern, the schemes finds families or individuals willing to be host to an old person who is not actually a relative or friend. The schemes are often promoted by voluntary organizations but local authorities can grant financial aid.

OUTPATIENT GERIATRICS

In chapter 3, I outlined the assessment of patients' needs at home through the visit by the hospital geriatrician. The patient whatever his or her age may be seen instead at the outpatient department of the geriatric unit; or be seen there following an initial home visit.

Outpatient departments vary a great deal from hospital to hospital and from area to area. One O.P.D. (as it is called for short) may be held in a draughty poorly-lit building with people huddled on long benches and winter heating a matter of frequent cups of tea. Another may be a modern purpose-built structure of glass and concrete with comfortable seating and central heating. The O.P.D. consultation rooms too may vary from a private interviewing room with two sound-proof cubicles off the sides, to an open twin-desked anteroom with curtain or hardboard cubicling through which all with ears must hear – all about as private as Euston station. The whole subject of the function, efficiency, and atmosphere of hospital outpatient departments has been investigated in a nation-wide survey by the Ministry of Health. Individual areas have been assessing their own problems and difficulties, both by time-and-motion study and research surveys.

The ideal geriatric outpatient department would be all on one level for easy reception of patients. Ancillary investigation departments should be near at hand, for example the pathology laboratory for blood tests and the X-ray department. At the present time, many geriatric O.P.D.s are up or down stairs from the receiving area and the ancillary departments are often a long walk or wheelchair ride away. Doctors consulting at a geriatric O.P.D. clinic operating under the latter disadvantage may take their own blood tests and even do their own X-ray screening where possible. But this means they have time to see fewer patients per session.

History-taking and examination anyway take longer with elderly outpatients than with others. As already mentioned, the older person is slower undressing, finds it harder to tell a coherent chronological story about the illness – or rather illnesses – tends to go off the point, and is slower at cooperating in a detailed clinical examination. Deafness which has not been corrected by hearing aid or trumpet or syringeing out ear wax adds to the general difficulties in some cases, as do other physical disabilities such as stiff limbs or creaky joints.

Since this is so, the number of old people to be seen in a given hour of O.P.D. clinic time should be less than in other specialties. Moreover nurses who are used to dealing swiftly and expeditiously with patients in other clinics, have to slow their pace and be ready to do much more explaining and helping. If the doctor has previously made a home visit and decided that the old person is fit to attend as an outpatient for blood tests, X-rays and other special examinations, he may then ask for subsequent O.P.D. attendances so that he can follow up. He tries to keep these to a minimum as even younger patients find frequent attendances tiring. Or he may send all the O.P.D. information to the family doctor (with whom he keeps in touch in any case) and advise on treatment and ask the family doctor to follow up instead. Of course, the O.P.D. findings may lead to a decision that hospital admission for further investigation or treatment is needed. Here again a preceding home visit can let the geriatrician judge social as well as medical priorities.

The previously mentioned 'ideal' geriatric O.P.D. would be adjacent to and continuous with the main unit, so that the outpatient could also be seen on the one visit by, say, the physiotherapists to assess need for exercises or short-wave therapy, or by the occupational therapist for recommendation of gadgets or re-educating in daily living activities. If the day hospital was also near, it could be shown to patients who might benefit from future attendance there, an improvement on the present 'try it once and see if you like it' method. Some geriatric units deny the need for any O.P.D. specially for the aged while others use it to replace or reinforce home visiting on a big scale, but most units have at least one O.P.D. clinic a week at present.

5

PREVENTIVE GERIATRICS

WE have already noted in chapter 4 the perspicacious remark of the health visitor who thought that the best time to teach and learn preventive (some prefer the term preventative) geriatrics was in middle age. This is the time when attention to health should pay dividends ten and twenty years later. The problem of what constitutes health, however, is much more difficult for the doctor – or any scientist for that matter – to define. Whereas disease processes can be defined in terms of their cause and effect, the state of health of a given individual might have to be outlined in terms of environment, childhood background, past and present social class, sex, actual chronological age, and social and personal habits.

A useful if rough good health guide-line runs along through the absence of any important physical symptoms or signs evident to the individual and an examining doctor, and the presence of a mental outlook which is forward-looking, confident, with a pride of purpose in life. As far as ageing is concerned, what the homespun philosophers tell us is essentially true – it is not years that count so much as the effect of physical and/or mental disease on the body growing older. (And should both these be operative and socio-economic circumstances poor as well, the human organism is under heavy fire indeed.)

A clearer definition of health in terms of the body systems, social class, age (by decades), and whether male or female, will emerge, as examining apparently healthy people as a 'routine' in commerce, industry, the professions and government services, becomes established. The U.S.A. promoted the idea on a big scale, in the higher echelons of commercial life, with the 'executives' check-up' which screened important men and women on their mental and physical state at regular intervals of, say, one year. These check-ups were carried out by the companies' own doctors or the family doctor or at recognized clinics. A similar but more centralized venture for executives in this country is the Medical Centre of the Institute of Directors.

The idea of preventive check-ups is also popular with the man – and woman – in the street, for all social classes have welcomed and supported such Public Health preventive measures as mass miniature radiography to detect tuberculosis, cervical smear tests for womb cancer in women, antivenereal disease campaigns, area screening tests in selected communities for hidden sugar diabetes, and the type of preventive clinic which we shall be looking at in the next part of this chapter. In fact the monies available for preventive services seem to be lagging behind the public demand.

Attention to the following points is worth a regular check in middle age, despite those pessimists who say we will breed a nation of introverted hypochondriacs if the National Health Service becomes less of a National Disease Service. Weight is the first and some would say the most important, and I shall be outlining the dangers and problems of obesity later in this chapter. Routine blood-pressure measurements can pinpoint the early and advancing hypertensives, who are so readily amenable to treatment today. Testing urine and blood samples will reveal hidden cases of sugar diabetes, kidney disease or anaemia – all treatable as a rule. X-ray of the chest picks out the bronchitics, to whom advice can be given on smoking, air pollution, and occupation. Tuberculosis and early lung cancer can also be detected and treatment initiated. Listening to the heart and doing an electro-cardiogram can show up potential heart troubles. Eye tests, ear tests and teeth inspection can all show whether there are appropriate measures to be taken. In men, prostate examination and in women, gynaecological examination can ensure abnormalities are treated. Advice on regular, reasonable exercise can be given and on the type of diet needed. Last but far from least, the mental state can be assessed and treatment and reassurance given.

PREVENTIVE CLINICS – THE RUTHERGLEN EXPERIMENT

In a country with a sound family doctor service, where there is no doctor shortage, where the doctor does not have to take on excess patients to keep his economy straight, where he can give as much time and attention to preventive medicine as to the treatment of disease – under such circumstances, the family doctor could see *healthy* middle-aged or ageing people to assess and check-up on physical, mental and social well-being. In the much less than ideal situation which existed before the inception of the National Health Service in 1948, and which the N.H.S. has but slightly remedied, the seed of an idea grew in the minds of many doctors, that a complementary screening set-up might be established either at the proposed health centres or at a special Public Health clinic.

The first seed germinated in Glasgow, Scotland, when in 1952, at the request of the local medical officer of health, the Secretary of State approved the setting up of the Rutherglen Consultative Health Centre for old people. The Rutherglen experiment, as it was called in those days, brought together the three wings of the N.H.S. – public health, hospital and family doctor services – to promote the health of the over-55s in the community. The age of 55 or over was taken as suitable for referral, and apparently healthy or possibly ill patients could be referred by their family doctor (only), on his initiative or at the patient's request, for a full diagnostic screening.

The first preventive clinic was staffed by the medical officer of health and the regional geriatrician, supported by health visitors and such ancillary personnel as physiotherapists, occupational therapists, chiropodists – with such diagnosing facilities as X-rays, electro-cardiograms and gynaecological department equipment available. A full medico-social assessment was made at the first visit, and a routine chest X-ray taken. The patient attended a second time for a clinical examination by the consultant geriatrician. Where illness or potential illness was found, the opinions and recommendations – for this was strictly an advisory service – were communicated to the family doctor. Such recommendations might include referral to the hospital geriatric unit or to another specialist – e.g. a general surgeon; or that the patient might be resettled in a welfare home; or administering of prophylactic antibiotics in the presence of chronic bronchitis; or . . . many other helpful ideas.

Where the referrals were found to be healthy over-55s, the clinic was able to collect important information on average measurements – height, chest expansion, upper and lower blood pressures, heart size, weight, and pulse rates. The relative sex incidence of diseases in the ill referrals – hypertension, arthritis, anaemia and so on – was also noted. In other words, such preventive clinics also have a useful research value for geriatrics and hence in the long run for community health.

As well as being an advice bureau for the over-55s, and a liaison advisory clinic for family doctors, the preventive clinic works closely with voluntary bodies who can provide other benefits and advice if the old person agrees to accept these. The clinics also help in the 'keep the patient at home' campaign, reducing the load on the hospital services.

The preventive clinics did not spread like wildfire as some

thought might happen, but they are gradually increasing in number. Some of the clinics have acted in a more direct welfare capacity by not just recommending but also providing vitamin supplements at low cost as a preventive measure, but caution is needed if the clinic is not to step out of its essentially advisory role and usurp the function of the patient's family doctor.

One of the important research findings of the original Rutherglen experiment was the high incidence of obesity in older women, and its deleterious effects on both sexes, but especially on men.

OBESITY – A SPECIAL PROBLEM

The effects on body health of being overweight are now regarded so seriously by doctors that the state of being more than 10 to 15 per cent overweight, i.e. obese, is regarded as a disease. While a relatively few cases of obesity are due to hormone disorders like lack of thyroid or too much cortisone, more than nine-tenths of cases of obesity are due to overeating. However vigorously fat people deny this, the essential reason for being overweight is that our regular eating habits involve our calorie (food) intake being always greater than our calorie (energy) output. Suitable calorie intakes for old people who want to keep their weight steady at a time of life when they tend to be less energetic, are discussed in the section on nutrition in chapter 7. The actuaries of insurance companies who calculate death risks, confirm the doctors' familiar statement that obesity shortens the expectation of life in both sexes, in middle age by up to a quarter. This killer effect is most marked in men, so that fat men rarely live to the ripe old age of their female counterparts.

A look at the illnesses and disabilities which are associated with obesity, makes us realize that, of all the preventive measures which we can take regarding future health, reduction of weight to normal levels for height and age is the most worthwhile. Overweight people are frequently short of breath because of the mechanical obstacles to the movements of respiration. As a consequence they are more likely to suffer from bronchitis and the risks of pneumonia as well as having difficulty with slopes and steps. Overweight persons are also more liable to high blood pressure and its secondary effects on the heart and the brain. The process of hardening of the arteries – known as atherosclerosis – is speeded up in obese people, causing such features as angina of effort and heart failure and poor circulation to the limbs. Obesity in old people is also significantly associated with diabetes (see p. 127).

Fat people are also likely to develop the 'wear and tear' of joints such as hips and knees known as osteoarthritis sooner than normal, and, in addition, run a greater risk of falls and subsequent broken limbs. The feet tend to flatten and ankles swell uncomfortably. When fat people become ill, they are more difficult to nurse and are especially liable to develop sores in the pressure areas of, for example, backs and heels.

Unfortunately, there is no universal psychologically acceptable method of weight reduction. In the first place, appeals to fashionable slimness are lost on the elderly, who do not put such high regard socially on an aesthetic appearance. Secondly, the old person is not at all keen to change a lifetime's habit of overeating or addiction to high calorie-value foods. Thirdly, eating may be a psychological bolster to a lonely or unhappy old person and advice on a reducing diet may provoke greater depression. Lastly, and this is so often the case in hospital, well-meaning relatives and friends bring food and drink in over-abundance when they visit the old person, and cajole them to enjoy part of it while the 'watchful eye' of nurse or doctor is out of range: a sort of being kind to be cruel.

Nevertheless, short-term admission to hospital may be

necessary to initiate a weight-reducing diet and ensure a substantial weight loss in the old person. There are no magic pills or potions which shed the superfluous fat. The standard medical diet for weight reduction is the low-calorie – 800 to 1,000 calories daily – diet which reduces starch, sugar and fat intake. As a psychological prop, patients may be given in addition to such diets, drugs that are said to reduce the appetite. The point to note is that appetite-reducing drugs by themselves – without a low-calorie diet – will not effectively reduce weight. Unfortunately many of these same drugs, especially those based on the amphetamine group, can cause drug dependence or addiction, if used for long periods. In any low-calorie diet and especially for elderly people, additional vitamins, iron and calcium may be prescribed.

As an alternative to normal low-calorie diets, the liquid or solid low-calorie 'formula' diet has appeared. This was first used on the other side of the Atlantic but has gained favour in the U.K., too. Short-term weight reduction is often reasonably successful but formula diets are often too expensive for fixed-income pensioners and, in any case, the artificial nature of this eating habit soon causes disenchantment and a return to the old ways.

The value of exercise in weight reduction is sometimes promoted but this is likely to increase a healthy appetite and, in elderly people, is not likely to be recommended in the presence of other disabilities. Hypnotic treatment with posthypnotic suggestion to support failing cases on low-calorie diets has been tried with varying success. Whether group therapy self-help treatment clubs, like Fatties Anonymous, will prove to be the answer, remains to be seen. In the meantime, hospital geriatric units, health visitors and preventive clinics must campaign vigorously, with the family doctors' full support, against the killer called obesity.

PREPARATION FOR RETIREMENT

I have already touched on the pre-retirement preparation theme in connexion with health, disease and obesity, but there are wider applications still. It is alarming how very many people reach retirement today with no real plan for its use and enjoyment, and no thought as to the socio-economic changes this salutary act may have. People talk vaguely of having more time to do the garden or go fishing or golfing, or of seeing the sights or having a nice long holiday; but the effect of coming home one day as the family bread-winner, a skilled employee, a favourite workmate, and waking up the next day as a fixed-income spouse, a retired employee, an ex-workmate who is already getting under his wife's feet at home, can bring resentment, depression, loss of purpose and mental disaster to the unprepared. Doctors and lay persons alike often quote how 'old so-and-so was fit as a fiddle in his job until he was forced to retire at 70, then he died in a few weeks after that'.

Two patterns have accentuated the problems of retirement in the present day. On the one hand the physical and mental health of persons in their sixties is much better than ever before. On the other, mechanization and automation and the fast pace of industrial and commercial life has steadily lowered compulsory retiral ages to 65, 60 or even 55. This means that skilled, trained and able people with good physical and mental capabilities, are being released into a leisure existence for which they are unprepared personally, for which there is inadequate community support, and which could last for a period of twenty to twenty-five years.

In the United States, where leisure time for all ages is greater than in the U.K., both commercial and industrial companies have organized pre-retirement courses (both internally and in association with local university colleges). Similarly, it was commercial concern in this country that initiated the first preparation-for-retirement programme. In 1958, the first representative Retirement Council – including commercial, trade union, industrial, medical, local authority and voluntary group members – was formed in Glasgow with the aims of studying the problems of the elderly worker and promoting education for retirement, promoting useful and diversionary retirement activities, and disseminating information and advice to all interested bodies or individuals.

The following year the Glasgow Retirement Council started day-release courses for older employees whose firms were agreeable to their attending without loss of earnings. The success of such courses will be measured over this and the coming decades but the pattern is obviously the right one, as retirement councils have sprung up far and wide nationally.

A suggested course of talks on planning for retirement, with the lecture given by an appropriate 'expert', and time allowed for study-discussion, might include the following items:

for men

1. retirement and money, to include information on retirement pensions, supplementary benefits, voluntary sources of help, and advice on organizing a suitable personal budget

2. retirement and physical health, to include advice on moderate exercise, the importance of fluids, diet and vitamins, attention to hearing, eyesight and teeth, and 'check-ups' from the family doctor

3. retirement and mental health, to include advice on mental exercise, limitations of mental vigour, importance of morale and forward outlook, value of companionship at home or in clubs, sexual problems

4. retirement and social living, to include notes on over-60s clubs, day centres, home services from the local authority,

meals-on-wheels, welfare holidays, adaptations of home, resettlement in other accommodation

5. retirement and leisure, to include notes on local and mobile libraries (with big-print books, and records), cinema and theatre and art galleries, crafts and hobbies and do-it-yourself activities, darts, bowls and other games, gardening, and – not quite 'leisure' – post-retirement part-time occupations

6. a discussion of the opportunities, value and consolations of age;

for women, a similar course of talks, but perhaps including under 5 charity and voluntary work, whist drives and – realistically – bingo.

In conjunction with such lecture-discussions, visits to the various places mentioned can be made, either literally or on film.

To me, some form of preparation for retirement seems as logical as mothercraft classes for school-leaver and antenatal women or apprentice night- and day-classes for workers in training. And this even though there are many people who already do prepare well and make the transition successfully without the elementary help outlined above.

VALUE OF THE GERIATRIC SURVEYS

Ever since the beginning of the National Health Service – and before for that matter – different groups or individuals have been carrying out surveys of the elderly community. Sociologists, economists, seekers after Ph.D. or M.D., physicians and geriatricians, local authority officers, medical officers of health and voluntary organization officers have all spent much time and effort to clarify the picture of the over-60s way of life. Sometimes they have concentrated on a narrow point like the level of vitamin deficiency, sometimes

on a broader problem like the question of suitable or unsuitable accommodation, sometimes on a wide front of
health, social and economic assessments. The point is that
only by going out 'into the field' can the current problems
and needs and the provisions and programme for the future
be delineated.

Prediction of social and medical needs in a given age group
is usually the function of the local authority health and
welfare departments at a local level and the Ministry of
Health and complementary departments of government at a
national level. For the elderly section of the population, both
home and hospital services will have to expand fairly rapidly
to meet the needs of the rising numbers mentioned in the
introduction to this book. The England and Wales hospital
plan* put the number of beds required in a geriatric unit –
of the kind already described – at 1·4 (beds can be 'split'
statistically) per 1,000 total population. Many areas have
reached or surpassed this figure, however, and find that they
still have a long waiting list with much pressure on beds.
A local geriatric survey would show the real need in each
area as opposed to an unrealistic 'average figure'.

From the local authority viewpoint, a local geriatric survey
can reveal not only the actual number of people waiting for
welfare home, flatlet or warden-supervised bungalow accommodation, but potential cases in the next few years, so that
the housing department can do forward purpose-building
planning. Local individual use of such services as district
nursing and home helps can also be checked, the potential
need for such services assessed, and plans for any necessary
expansion of the departments formulated.

On a strictly medical level, hidden cases of illness like
anaemia, arthritis and foot defects can be brought to light,
and a full picture obtained of the incidence of disabilities

* *A Hospital Plan for England and Wales*, H.M.S.O., 1962, Cmnd
1604.

like poor vision, unsteadiness, deafness and slowness of movement. This in turn can bring all the medical, nursing, social and voluntary services already discussed into play. Psychiatric problems such as apathy, depression, paranoia, personality degeneration, mental confusion can also be brought out, and the interplay of these with the physical and socio-economic state studied so that they can be tackled on the hospital and hostel and services pattern. Surveys also reveal how effective current deployment of staff and services are in the preventive geriatric scheme, and what immediate steps can be taken to improve or alter the situation.

All surveys are time-consuming, and facts which can be ascertained by simple reference to, say, family doctor records or the Census should be excluded. Modern computer-programming of survey data can be used for forward planning and rapid current assessment in the geriatric sphere.

6

VOLUNTARY WORK IN GERIATRICS

It is a familiar pattern in the English way of life that where there is a social problem, private individuals working alone or in groups will voluntarily take up the matter and work out a solution. Further, they will seek charitable or other voluntary financial assistance to set the solution in motion and then, when it is demonstrably effective, local or national statutory help will be forthcoming. This has been the story with help for physically handicapped children, mentally handicapped children and adults, blind and deaf adults and others. This has also been the pattern with the problems and social needs of the elderly community.

Long before the pioneers of geriatric medicine were evolving their new methods and approach, local groups in town and county were aware of the difficulties, handicaps and hardships of the elderly, and organizing manual, financial and other practical help under the central patronage of the National Council of Social Service. The Second World War exacerbated the difficulties of the elderly in the community, and it was realized that a specific central group to deal with matters affecting the elderly was urgently required. Thus, in 1940, the National Old People's Welfare Committee came into being, as a coordinating body of all groups interested in helping the elderly. Like the doctors' Society, it underwent a change of name – in 1955, to National Old People's Welfare Council, by which name it is still known and under whose banner are represented local old people's welfare committees, numerous other voluntary associations, government departments and local authority associations.

Despite the government department representatives, the Council is apolitical and independent, with the Social Service National Council as its trustees. On a national level, the value of such a Council representing the needs of a previously low-priority group like the elderly is tremendous. It can effectively coordinate opinions and advice on major issues for the elderly, such as national and local housing policies, the needs for home services in different areas, and important schemes like night attendance provision, lunch clubs and chiropody. It publishes a quarterly journal with the news and views of its constituent members and manages to retain some of the pioneering spirit with which it all began. Advice and suggestions on practical problems are made available locally and nationally, and there is good liaison at the local level with welfare departments and geriatric units and the family doctor service.

Most voluntary organizations working on a national scale have found it necessary to have paid part-time and full-time officers, in order to provide a round-the-clock comprehensive and efficient service. With trained people in the key positions, voluntary work in the field of old age can be channelled in the right paths, and duplication with thin spreading avoided. I use the agricultural analogy for voluntary work is, after all, down to earth.

The Council was originally self-financing through voluntary appeals, and monies still come from well-wishers and 'charity functions'. Help financially also came in the 1950s from the National Corporation for the Care of Old People. The latter was founded in 1947 when funds from the Nuffield Foundation – a pioneer in geriatric surveys – were joined with the Air Raid Distress Fund to create an independent Corporation. Its stated aims are to finance research into problems of the elderly, to study the changing needs of the elderly, and to support by grant and loan groups or organizations or individuals carrying out such functions.

In the course of this book I have already touched upon many of the services which the voluntary groups like the old people's welfare committees can and do initiate, organize, sponsor and promote. Apart from effectively publicizing the needs of the elderly at conferences or seminars, they may organize leisure and lunch clubs, old people's outings and the requisite transport, individual services like shopping, decorating, home reading, repairs; arrange holidays, night or day visiting, spiritual activities; support mobile meals and library services; help with boarding out schemes; make recommendations for welfare homes; ensure advice on aids and adaptations ... assist indeed with the whole gamut of old people's requirements, other than the purely medical, at any time.

W.R.V.S. – MEALS-ON-WHEELS

Lest any member take umbrage at the opening initials, I should remind you that this important voluntary group is now the Women's Royal Voluntary Service. These familiar green-clothed ladies play a distinguished role in the voluntary services provided for old people. In hospitals, the mobile library and the mobile stationery and sweet shops are seen at all times of the day bringing pleasure to patients and to many of the staff, too. Before the advent of official occupational therapy departments, they provided – often still do – diversional amenities such as knitting, tatting, embroidery and hand games like dominoes and draughts.

In 1941, the W.V.S. as it then was, in parallel with several other voluntary organizations, set up residential homes for the elderly in need of care and attention. These homes continue to flourish and new ones are opened from time to time. Local authorities are, in a limited way, able to help with costs for some of the residents if, for example, their own welfare vacancies are all full.

The W.R.V.S. is the largest provider of home meals for the elderly, serving several million hot meals yearly. I shall be dealing with nutrition in the elderly in the next chapter, but the meals-on-wheels service is an important corrective of undernourishment and dietary imbalance. The scheme supplies by arrangement a hot meal at an economical price to the old person's own home, as near midday as is feasible. The meals are carried in cars or vans or, in outlying areas, partly on foot, in heat-retaining containers, having been cooked at a local meals centre or by voluntary cooks or even at a factory canteen. The cars and vans may be W.R.V.S. members' own or loaned.

The service can only supply a small percentage of the elderly, and then not more than twice a week as a rule. Many local authorities are now giving grants towards capital or running costs or both, but the potential of such a service is enormous, and not yet being properly exploited.

Another W.R.V.S. promotional venture is the setting up of clubs for the elderly and supporting their running and activities. The W.R.V.S. is also responsible for organizing lecture courses and study–discussion groups which train and direct their own members and other voluntary workers.

It would be invidious to single out the W.R.V.S. and not mention the parallel work of setting up homes, providing meals-on-wheels, organizing elderly persons' clubs and training voluntary workers which the British Red Cross and its associated societies undertake on a large scale. They also have local medical loan depots supplying bed pans, rubber bed sheets, various types of wheelchair, back-rests and other forms of nursing equipment for the elderly sick. They are also famous for their pen friends promotion scheme for hospital patients.

This is not, and cannot be, a comprehensive handbook of

voluntary organizations for the elderly. I can only apologize for the omission of all the names of the leagues, societies and helpers of old people that do not appear in any of the chapters. They know how important their work is to the elderly and that is what counts.

OVER-60S CLUBS

There is an apocryphal story of a glamorous grandmother of 70 who admitted she enjoyed other people's company but rarely left her own four walls and the cat. When asked why she didn't join the local over-60s club, she told the voluntary worker that she couldn't bring herself to go along and reveal her real age to her neighbours.

Fortunately, few elderly people are as acutely sensitive about their age as that lady and most welcome the provision of clubs of a voluntary nature, whose activities are geared to the older population. In the big conurbations, day clubs have grown rapidly in number in the last ten years to serve local areas. The value of the club as a meeting place for local old people with similar backgrounds and similar interests lies in several directions. It encourages people to participate in group activities instead of apathetically ruminating in the loneliness of solitude. It provides a positive event to look forward to, in a daily life which otherwise may tend to an unappetizing sameness. It fosters a sense of belonging and pride in one's community. It gives opportunity for continued self-expression through self-help and helping other members of the club.

Whether the club is run for one afternoon a week or open daily, will depend on the demand from its members, the availability of the premises if they are hired or on loan, and the support of its initiators – the old people's welfare committee, W.R.V.S., Red Cross or other voluntary workers and groups. Some groups have managed to buy their own premises through fund-raising 'charity functions' and private benefactions, and so have them continuously available. The club may have an organizer from one of the voluntary groups, or an internal club member may take the job on; in any case, all members are encouraged to participate in the organizing of daily and special activities. Making the tea, arranging a birthday party, decorating the walls, acting as hostess to visitors or new members, promoting club outings ... the opportunity for active participation is always there. Retired people with special skills like joinery, upholstery, hairdressing or flower-arranging are encouraged to do-it-themselves and help others to inside the club.

Clubs which provide a meal, or lunch and afternoon tea, are useful in combating the indifferent nutrition of many old people. Specified luncheon clubs can offset their costs by aid from local authorities as well as by the small sums paid by the diners. Clubs may 'specialize' in particular attractions, such as folk-dancing or choir singing, or keep-fit classes or drama or concerts. Film nights or rather film afternoons, lectures from 'specialist' community workers like health visitors and doctors, more general talks, slide shows, indoor and some outdoor games, are all part of the mixture of social entertainment and cultural pleasure at the clubs.

From the geriatrics viewpoint, the register of members kept by the club can be most valuable. Members know, for example, who has not been turning up lately, and arrangements can be made for sick visiting and notifying the member's family doctor and the home services. Thus old people living alone do not have to wait until some observant neighbour in the street wonders why eight bottles of milk outside Mrs A's are still full and uncollected, before help is forthcoming. The clubs can also give moral support to their members in times of stress, such as family loss.

Clubs of a different membership, based on disability or infirmity, have been established. These day centres, as they are called, have already been outlined in chapter 4, when I was discussing how their function contrasts with that of the day hospital. Some local authorities have used the organization, facilities and staff of residential homes to set up small day centres for the local disabled elderly.

Another Glasgow innovation some years ago was the idea of retired employee's associations, where workers who had retired from the same company or works, could meet together in a suitable hall for similar activities to the ones already described for over-60s clubs. Professional retired people also have societies for their own needs, and golf clubs and Masonic groups share the company of senior businessmen as well. Religious groups have their own clubs for denominational members, again with a varied programme of events. The wide range of over-60s clubs should mean that all sections of the elderly community are catered for, and could mean that the old person can be a member of two, three and more clubs if he or she is up to it.

OTHER GROUPS – e.g. ROUND TABLE, CHURCH GUILDS, SIXTH-FORMERS

There are many other groups who actively help their local elderly people – young people (under 40) like those of the Round Table who run, for example, Christmas hamper or winter coal schemes; young and middle-aged people (under 60) like members of church guilds who run bus outings to the seaside or Christmas parties, or 'Sound of Music' visits; young people (under 20) like sixth-formers who run hospital visiting 'adoption' or home decoration help schemes. Healthy and fully independent over-60s also aid and support less fortunate contemporaries in the same senior age group.

In fact, wherever people get together in groups, there will always be some positive individual who will say 'Let's do something for our old people', and another venture in voluntary geriatric work is under way. There is a continuing need for such activity, as the elderly community grows and the family-unit system breaks up leaving more old people on their own. Of course all activities of this kind are even more effective if there is cooperation and coordination in any given community, and this is where the local representatives of the National Old People's Welfare Council can help.

CHEAP SERVICES – e.g. CINEMAS, HAIRDRESSING, TRANSPORT

The obvious fact that old people have to live on a fixed income has encouraged a social conscience in certain commercial groups, whether maintained by private enterprise or rate-payers. These groups provide cheap, or more correctly cheaper, services for people who can show evidence of belonging to the elderly community, such as a pension book or over-60s club card. Some cinema circuits provide cheaper seats for over-60s either at matinees or on certain evenings of the week. Men's and women's hairdressers encourage hygiene and an interest in personal appearance by reducing prices for 'short back and sides' or 'perms' to all pensioners.

Many corporation transport departments offer a cheap rate at certain periods for travelling pensioners. A scheme bringing fares within old people's reach is invaluable. And if it operates, say, between ten and four on weekdays, this allows them time to visit relatives or friends or sick people in hospital, or to attend the day clubs we have discussed above.

Other concerns, such as shops, cafés, markets, may offer discounts to pensioners. Not every old person likes the idea of a sort of 'charitable treatment', but in the face of a steadily rising cost of living, very many take advantage of the concessions to eke out their current retirement pension.

Cheap accommodation is a different matter. (For something of old people's difficulties with housing costs see the next chapter, page 102.) Temporary cheap accommodation is available at local authority model lodging houses, but the overseers do not allow their temporary residents to lie abed by day. The Salvation Army through its hostels provides shelter for old people, often of the nomadic variety, but including also 'home-grown' poor who would otherwise sleep 'rough'. But the Army insists on its residents being up out of bed by day, which leads to difficulties in short-term illnesses (in any age group). The Salvationists do in fact nurse their wards temporarily but signs of need for more prolonged medical and nursing care will lead to a call from the G.P. attending the Salvation Army hostel to, where the sick person is elderly, the hospital's geriatrician. Prisons too have their share of the poorer elderly seeking refuge and 'cheap accommodation', particularly recidivists of waning powers and low-I.Q. unfortunates. The story of the old man at Christmas, breaking a window so the magistrate will send him to a warm 'free' cell and 'free' pudding, is not fictitious.

7

OTHER SOCIAL AND ECONOMIC ASPECTS

ROLE OF THE MEDICAL SOCIAL WORKER

I HAVE already indicated in chapter 2 that the hospital's medical social worker, sometimes called M.S.W. for short, is a member of the geriatric 'team'. Moreover she is an absolutely invaluable member whose work ties up the many strands of information, advice, therapy and outlook for patients, before, during and after their progress through the hospital's geriatric unit. The name medical social worker replaces the previously familiar title of 'lady almoner', with its past associations of collections and disbursement of hospital monies for the poor sick attending hospitals. The change to M.S.W. followed the decision of the Institute of Almoners to set behind it the long history of almoning, from the appointment of Mary Stewart to the Royal Free Hospital in 1895 at the instigation of the Charity Organization Society, through to 1922 when the Institute of Hospital Almoners was established. Following the Royal College of Physicians Report of 1943 on the function of almoners (assessment of the patients' needs not the patients' means) the profession was brought right up to date in its medical social role extending from the hospital into the community.

There can be no question that the hospital's geriatric unit, of all the specialist departments, puts the heaviest work load on the M.S.W. department. Where possible therefore, geriatric units welcome a full-time M.S.W. for the department, but most often they can call only part-time on the services of these helpful ladies, who are ever in short supply. Most old people coming into the unit are likely to need and be seen and helped by the M.S.W. at some time in their illness.

Doctors pride themselves on being good listeners (though patients do not always agree with this self-assessment) but no one, except perhaps a psychiatrist, knows how to listen in such a positive manner as the M.S.W. As she listens to the patient or the relatives, she notes details of personal and social history; interpersonal relationships; mood and feelings; attitudes towards money, family, illness, job; positive or negative outlook; moral and ethical attributes; cultural and intellectual levels. With such a broad picture of her interviewee, she can then apply her social training in the most helpful and realistic direction, supporting the medical and rehabilitation therapy and paving the way for the patient's return to an active life on the socio-economic level.

By letter, telephone, personal interview, inter-staff meetings, round-table conferences, working lunches and the like, the M.S.W. acts as a vital liaison link between the other members of the 'team', the patient, relatives, friends and neighbours, the local authority departments, voluntary groups, ambulance service and . . . anyone or any body concerned with her patient-contact. Thus practical measures, like ensuring that the patient's home or welfare home place is not given up, or that bills are regularly paid, or that a pension is drawn and benefits understood, or that the house is warmed and food is available for the homecomer, or relatives forewarned, and all concerned know about home services – all this and more is part of the M.S.W.'s work.

Just as valuable for the smoother progress from hospital back home, is the M.S.W.'s capacity to correct, modify or dispel false premisses or notions and unrealistic attitudes in both relatives and patients. With limitless patience, courtesy, kindness, wit, and in the privacy of an interview room, she can guide people in a better direction and enlist help from

previously untapped or unapproachable sources. A geriatrician might paraphrase the best known Englishman with
'Give me an M.S.W. and I'll finish the job.'

RETIREMENT AND SUPPLEMENTARY PENSIONS

Frequently in the preceding chapters, I have stressed that
the elderly community is for the most part a fixed-income
group. This implies financial lack of elasticity to meet the
steady rise in the cost of living (e.g. by doing overtime or
bonus work), to meet inflation (e.g. by earning interest
on capital or profits on insurance policies); hence to afford
regular replacement of clothes, footwear, furnishings,
decoration, worn appliances, or desirable extras (called
luxuries) such as holidays, 'nights out', sweets and tobacco,
birthday gifts and the like.

Old-age pensions or, more correctly, retirement pensions
can be claimed from the Ministry of Social Security (the
subtly renamed former Ministry of Pensions and National
Insurance) at any age between 65 and 70 after retirement from
regular employment. Women are entitled to claim between
60 and 65.

Unhappily, state retirement pensions have been a re-
curring political carrot in the policies of all parties over
very many years. No real attempt has been made to link the
flat-rate retirement pension to the rising cost of living.
Politicians of all parties point to the steady rise in such
pensions under either Right or Left, but ignore the effect of
inflation on the real value of the actual cash to the old person.
Even today's retirement flat-rate pension (due to be raised
by 10s. at the time of writing) of £4 a week plus £2 16s.
for a wife as dependant, compares ludicrously with a teen-
ager's pocket money of say £3 a week. Of course, the
guaranteed level for a retirement pension is higher at £4 15s.
for a householder or £7 10s. for a householding married

couple plus provision for rent (£4 10s. including provision for rent, for a non-householder) and application to the Ministry for supplementary pension to bring the basic level up to the guaranteed level can ensure a slightly improved financial state.

The old non-graduated contributory retirement pension was based on National Insurance contributions over the years, an arrangement which produced a flat-rate retirement pension that did not really take account of the actual pre-retirement level of income and resultant pre-retirement standard of living of the individual concerned. It may be that the graduated contributory pension scheme and many superannuation schemes will mean many future members of the elderly community are at less of a disadvantage financially. (And the existence of the state graduated pension scheme will not preclude those who will not benefit, having earned poorly all their lives, getting Supplementary Benefit.) Old people, even so, are not always the best administrators of their own budget. Some will not modify lifetime habits of buying the best or newest product, while others are swayed by high-pressure salesmanship or cunning advertising into excessive or unnecessary purchasing.

Careful pre-retirement assessment of finance, as we have noted in chapter 5, is the basis of at least some success in coping with the problems of making ends meet in retirement. It should prevent the kind of situation I have seen arise – the thin undernourished shivering old lady, brought into Casualty nearly dead and suffering from exposure and starvation, who had been living on the basic pension although she had several thousand pounds in £5 notes stuffed in an old mattress; the unhappy dejected old man who was found outside the doors of a welfare department, deposited there by the owners of a nursing home who discovered the man had used all his life savings capital and still owed them three weeks back fees; the genteel old lady who refused financial help from the old National Assistance Board ('I would never take charity, young man') and material help from the home help and district nurse departments, and was eventually brought into hospital (under a compulsory order) with incontinence, itching, hair lice, and unbelievably malodorous and caked clothing and underwear, complaining that she didn't want to be with working-class inmates. Of course, these are extreme examples; plenty of retired people have made ample provision for income in later years, which they use wisely.

The Supplementary Benefits Commission, which has replaced the old National Assistance Board, can provide an old person with a pension where the necessary contributions were never actually paid. It can give help towards an old person's rent or rates and make special allowances for special diets, as for instance for diabetics. Where National Health Services are chargeable for, as say with dentures and spectacles, it can make refunds. Emergency needs such as, say, extra fuel and blankets in severe weather, can be met by the Commission promptly. An officer of the Commission will visit promptly on receipt of a special form obtained from any Post Office. (A neighbour, relative or friend can obtain the form and post it for the old person, of course.)

The difference between a basic and a comfortable way of life is one of the fuels that stoke the fires of ambition in younger men. Whether or not living on the poverty borderline encourages illness through poor food or not enough of it, inadequate clothes and room-heating, and insufficient social and mental stimulus, there seems no doubt that a better-fed, better-clothed, better-warmed, better-stimulated old person, such as the welfare home resident, can withstand disease and stress just that bit better. The remedy is not to advise all people over 60 to go into welfare homes but to set a better all-round standard of living for the elderly community.

One of the greatest millstones depressing that standard is,

precisely, the cost of housing. For all the new alertness to the needs old people's housing should, ideally, meet, and the efforts local authorities and voluntary bodies have been making to make approximations to the ideal available at less than market-economic rent (see pages 72–3), *the* major problem for countless elderly folk today is still affording a roof – any kind of roof. Subsidized rents and rate rebates in council housing may be helpful to old people already council tenants. Rents for newer special housing, such as old people's bungalows or parts of estates modified for the elderly, may be fairly low compared with average levels in the general community, but dear to an old person coming from a low-rent property demolished in slum clearance. The bedsitting-room, beloved of stage and TV playwrights, is a familiar urban pattern for cheap living, and sometimes old houses bought up cheaply by 'non-developers' have been turned into rabbit-warrens of 'bed-sits' for poorer old people. Widows, bachelors and spinsters especially gravitate to such accommodation, often to pay excessive rents for the privileges of drab social isolation and still less in the 'housekeeping' kitty. As things are, all one can do to help is often to make sure they know about the Supplementary Benefits Commission – which probably helps nutritionally, but not much to make life more worth keeping fit for.

Thrifty individuals who have accumulated a goodly sum in savings and insurance, and those old people who can still do a part-time job, can be better off than their absolutely-fixed-income contemporaries. But one cannot blame a victim of the great Depression or someone severely disabled for not having put himself into either of the two former categories. A welfare state must be prepared to act so that we do not have cheerful, well-nourished, forward-looking, materially well-off teenagers at one end of life and apathetic, undernourished, backward-looking, materially badly off pensioners at the distal end.

SHELTERED WORKSHOPS

The employment problems of elderly men have been and still are being studied, both at national and local level. Several bigger and some smaller industrial and other concerns have given a lead by introducing part-time schemes for older employees and redeployment to less tiring or less intensive work.

Traditionally, the older man has found himself night-watchman at his brazier, letter-bearer and tea-maker, sweeper-up–washer-down. No elderly employee who has been a skilled artisan or fine craftsman or semi-skilled worker, can relish such menial tasks, even as the basis of continued employment. The sheltered workshop, where elderly men could either make items at nominal rates of pay or just enjoy using their old work tools, tables, lathes, etc., to produce non-saleable items for pleasure and mental stimulus, was an idea pioneered by one of the old London borough councils and taken up at many centres of industry throughout the country. Whether the workshop is financially self-supporting, through being tied to a commodity outlet, or grant-aided by local authorities, the physical and psychological outlook of the old people so 'employed' is vastly improved. Complementary schemes for women have also been tried successfully in some places. The term 'sheltered' is used as an indication that the elderly men and women are not expected to undertake regular employment under normal working conditions and for normal working hours, because of the effect of their age and attendant minor or major disabilities.

Such workshops are not the whole answer to re-employing elderly people who are keen to do a job despite their enforced retirement. The interest of the Ministry of Labour in the general problem of ageing and employment, coupled with the changing pattern of the needs of the elderly in the community, may stimulate other useful solutions for the future. This applies not only to workers in industry but to former executives and former professional men.

RELATIVES' AND FRIENDS' SUPPORT

It took a catastrophic childhood death rate, and mammoth early crippledom, in the eighteenth and early nineteenth centuries, to awaken national interest in the prevention and treatment of childhood illness. This resulted in the development of a public health programme for ante-natal and maternal education. The sympathy which a crippled child evokes in an adult mind is not necessarily matched by similar emotions towards an elderly disabled person. The disastrous sentiment, 'Well, she's had her day', is a commoner evocation. Such a negative thought is a reflection of the compartmentalized approach to life in this twentieth century – childhood, teenage, middle age, old age. We often fail to view the individual life as a decade-to-decade progression, with each phase influencing the next. Any medical or social programme that sets out to change the pattern of care for and public services' approach to the elderly section of the population, will need to take account of the non-professionally involved section of the community and interest and advise them and support their efforts.

Relatives of old people are not a homogeneous group. The changing pattern of family life – from the larger Victorian family with at least one spinster daughter who stayed home and tended mama and papa, to the smaller modern family with the working wife or daughter – has reduced the number of potential attendant relatives. Since women outlive men by an average four or five years, an elderly man quite often has an elderly wife to care for him but the elderly woman is more likely to be widowed or a spinster. Brothers or sisters are apt to be elderly themselves and often still in the grip of family intolerance, unready or unwilling to join forces when help is needed. Children live away from their elders, both sexes are employed, they have their own families to attend to, and may expect 'the state' to take over moral and physical responsibility for their old parents. A kind of Parkinson's Law applies in some families, where the greater the number of offspring, the fewer available to help the elders. Often, the continued support of an old person falls steadily on one relative's broad shoulders with only minor support from the others. The reverse of the coin is sometimes seen, where grandchildren or cousins or nieces and nephews take in or help the old person 'for pity's sake' when closer relatives refuse to help or have died. Nevertheless, close relatives are still a main support for old people, in times of illness or when they become frail and more dependent on others.

The personality, habits, moods and needs of old people run through the whole spectrum of human nature: from the narrow, self-centred, obsessive and domineering to the broad-minded, philanthropic, expansive and can't-do-enough-to-help-you. Since relatives themselves have their own make-up, whether they and their elderly charges will have good rapport depends on the clash or matching of their respective interests and outlooks. Nevertheless, even the best, most harmonious relationships may be strained at times. This strain may be all the greater if sickness, paralysis, falls, incontinence or forgetfulness, for example, produce a load which the relatives are not trained to cope with or have not been given advice on tackling.

At times of strain, the relatives may press the family doctor for admission of the old person to the geriatric unit. The hospital geriatrician on his assessment visit may or may not agree that admission to hospital is required. This may produce a clash between the service provided by the hospital (which must be broadly helpful to as many old people as possible) and the immediate desires of the relative (which are necessarily individual and short-term). The introduction of skilled services like the district nurse and help schemes like home help and laundry services, with the offer of short-term admission for 'holiday-relief' at a later date (usually in the less-pressed summer months) may resolve the situation.

Some relatives are instinctively good with their old people, encouraging self-help, self-movement and self-sufficiency – in dressing, washing, cleaning, cooking, etc. – however slow their actions seem to the younger onlooker and however delaying to the daily schedule. Other relatives fuss, molly-coddle and cocoon their elderly, reducing their independence to a minimum or even keeping them mostly in bed, where 'they are safer' or 'won't get in the way'.

Many old people who live alone depend on the assistance of kind friends and neighbours. The closer the community – a small, distinct village, say, or a terrace 'row' of houses – the greater the contact among neighbours and the better the care prospects for a frail or bed-bound old person. In multi-storey flats, purpose-built bungalows or new estates the neighbourly instinct is apt to lapse, and there is less spontaneous community support of old people.

I have twice recalled our health visitor who recommended the 'un-teaching' of preconceived notions on the care of the elderly. Relatives and neighbours may not take kindly to advice, but it can benefit their elderly charges inestimably if they can be persuaded, for instance, to encourage even frail old folk to sit out and walk a few steps daily; arrange for hearing aids and new spectacles instead of accepting deafness and poor vision as 'inevitable'; insist that clothes and not night apparel, and shoes, not slippers, are worn daily; help ill patients to the commode or turn them over or lift them up in bed as the trained adviser can show them; give rehabilitated 'stroke' or arthritic cases only the necessary help with feeding or getting about ... just a few of the things which can mean the difference between an almost independent 80-year-old and a heavily dependent 70-year-old.

NUTRITION

I have already discussed one aspect of nutrition in the elderly. This was over-nutrition and the production of obesity with its attendant disabilities and body system disturbances and 'killer effect' in men. The point about reducing weight by eating less food (calories) than needed for energy output (also measured in calories) was forcefully made.

In old people generally, it would be expected that the total food requirement to keep at a steady weight – without developing either obesity or malnutrition – would be less, in terms of calories, than for the younger population. Since work ceases on retirement – or is reduced in late working life – and since housework and domestic duties are also lessened, the total energy output is less and the intake required less. Some have suggested that the rate at which the body organs and cells work (body metabolism) is slower in old age and hence fuel needs less, but this has not really been proved.

An average intake of between 2,000 and 2,500 calories daily, representing about one third less than for the adult worker or housewife, is considered about right for most old people. The total calories would need to be correspondingly increased if part-time work or more strenuous domestic duties were carried on. The popular notion that old people take their calories mostly as bread and jam sandwiches with sweet tea, or fish and chips with peas from the corner shop, is not borne out by several surveys of the eating habits of the elderly population. Certainly, up to the mid-70s, elderly women maintain well-balanced diets made up of varied cooked and ready-served foods. The balance often suffers, however, as they move into their eighties and become increasingly dependent on others.

Many elderly men depend for meals on cooking by female relatives, friends and neighbours, or on 'bought and brought in' food. Even when they do really cook for themselves, they tend to have less variety and, in particular, omit vitamin C-containing foods, or mis-cook them. Of all vitamin deficiencies in the elderly, the commonest in both sexes is lack of vitamin C. The vitamin is present in fresh fruit and canned fresh fruit juice, green vegetables, tomatoes and potatoes. Unfortunately the vitamin C is readily destroyed by heat so that overcooking removes it. Vitamin C is needed for keeping the body 'supporting tissue' healthy and helping wounds to heal, and lack of it causes scurvy. If an old person lacks the vitamin and cannot afford fresh fruit or fresh fruit juices, his doctor can give him pure vitamin C in tablet form.

The idea that the blood gets 'thinner' as we grow older is a popular misconception based on the frequency of anaemia in old people. The commonest anaemia is due to lack of iron in the diet and particularly affects women. Such good iron-containing foods as liver and kidneys as well as eggs and corned beef are popular with old people, and not so expensive as to be out of their reach, although the individual budget may limit the amount taken. Bread and potatoes are poorer sources of iron but do have a little to help them along. Severe iron deficiency needs doctor's iron tablets or injections or even transfusion in hospital.

Old people are also advised to have plenty of protein foods such as meat, eggs, fish and milk. Again the individual budget may limit such protein-rich foods, which are needed as cell builders, particularly after the stress of operations or illness. Unfortunately, synthetic protein-rich powders which can be prescribed in hospital after such stress, are classed as 'foods' outside in the community and not prescribable by family doctors.

Recent work has shown that the bone thinning, called osteoporosis, which is a feature of ageing may be due to lack of calcium and phosphorus in the diet. This should be fairly readily corrected by following the advertising advice to drink an extra pint of milk a day. This is important, as thin bones are more liable to break on falling, producing fractured hips or shoulders, for example.

We have already noted that luncheon clubs and meals-on-wheels can help to prevent food deficiencies in old people, though these services need much expansion. In certain cases, too, the Supplementary Benefits Commission can give extra allowances for special foods – to diabetics, for example. Despite this, geriatric units see cases of malnutrition not infrequently through the year. The patients may be suffering from physical disease which is debilitating, or mental disease which prevents them purchasing, cooking and regularly eating, or weakness and loss of appetite from loneliness and depression, or insufficient food through poverty and failure to apply for supplementary benefits. These patients may be admitted in a dying state and are particularly at risk to pneumonia, pressure sores and clots in the lung even in hospital. Reversal of the malnourished state by intravenous or stomach-tube feeding and multi-vitamin injection is not always successful if there is underlying organ disease, but is usually attempted and may be encouragingly worthwhile.

There are other problems of feeding which arise from the dentures that most old people have acquired. Some have ill-fitting or cracked sets which hurt them so that they take them out to eat; others can cope with and enjoy most foods with dentures in place but find their 'helpers' cutting up all the food beforehand. People with bad teeth, or lacking any, should be encouraged to see the dentist for dentures and then to wear them all the time. Fads and dislikes about food mature and solidify with age and no amount of cajoling, explaining or pleading by relatives, friends or professional workers will change the 'I never touch' brigade. Any likely vitamin or mineral deficiencies in this group just have to be assessed and corrected by medication.

AN ETHICAL QUESTION

From time to time, letters and articles appear in the national and local press and in the various magazines, concerning old people and their medical treatment. Often the writer has an elderly relative – say, mother or aunt – suffering from physical or mental disabilities which have reduced her to a state of extreme dependence on her attendants, or alternatively which have resulted in a loss of contact with realities and erased recognition of familiar people and loved ones. The naturally distressed observer writes an emotionally charged letter, condemning medical men for injudicious use of the drugs and modern therapy which keep such patients alive. It is suggested that the doctors should hold their hand if an illness, such as pneumonia, that could end the patient's twilight life, appears.

An attitude of this sort in relatives or friends who have known the patient in the prime of life, and at his or her fullest powers, and who now observe a shadow of the former personality in the hospital bed or armchair – such a 'wouldn't he (or she) be better off out of it all?' attitude is well understood by doctors and nurses in geriatrics. It is easier for professional attendants, who have never known the 'other' person, to accept this disabled human being as he or she is, and nurse and treat him or her as a whole person however organically damaged. In the community of the hospital, it would be invidious to single out patients for rejection of care and therapy, simply on the basis of 'they are no use to themselves or others', and a gross misplacement of the trust that all ill people – sophisticated or simple, old or young – place in the medical and nursing profession.

While doctors no longer take the original Hippocratic oath, many medical schools ask their doctors to take a simple oath, just before graduation. This usually involves a proclamation that the graduand will fulfil his obligations to heal the sick and relieve pain and suffering wherever and whenever possible. It does not specify any conditions for applying these principles nor does it qualify them by suggesting that because a patient is sub-intelligent, backward, antisocial, very old, unpleasant to look at, bed-bound, incurable or immoral, then the doctor must forgo applying his medical skill.

It is true that society today is placing more and more social decisions on the doctors' doorstep. Decisions on therapeutic abortion, decisions on dangerous drugs and addicts, decisions on who shall have the use of scarce artificial kidney machines, decisions on who shall have intensive cardiac treatment though apparently moribund – these are judgements the traditional scientific and dogmatic teaching of the medical schools does not really equip students to make. Doctors on the other hand are loath to pass these problems on to the lay committees and administrators who control hospital policy and progress. Perhaps the General Medical Council, or an extension of it, will lead the medical profession in pointing the path for doctors in their personal responsibilities to their patients.

In the meantime, as far as geriatric patients are concerned, anything remotely resembling euthanasia must be briskly rebuffed and countered by explanation and discussion with the relatives and friends concerned. In many cases, the reason that friends and relatives do rush into print, or air their grievances in TV and radio discussion programmes, is lack of communication with the specialists and nurses and doctors responsible for the particular old person. Geriatricians as a rule do try and make time for seeing relatives and are ever ready to talk about their mutual interest – the elderly patient. In most hospitals it is only a question of relatives asking for an explanatory interview, for it to be granted.

SEX

In a society like our own, which equates youthfulness with sexual vigour and ageing with impotence and absence of sexual activity, the question of sex in the sixth and seventh decades is generally treated depreciatively or casually dismissed. Even though sex matters are freely discussed in social conversation and all aspects of sexual function permeate the mass media of radio, TV, cinema, and the press, it is still apparently taboo for elderly citizens to imply or hint that this psycho-physical need is still a part of their lives. Elderly men, in particular, who express an interest in physical matters affecting the opposite sex are readily labelled with the epithet 'dirty old man'. The idea that sexual needs and activity slacken after middle age is a reasonable assumption, but the tacitly accepted viewpoint that arriving at a given age, for example at the change of life or at retirement from employment, means automatic cessation of desire and function is untrue and calls for much re-appraisal.

Sexologists often draw attention to great men who admitted to sexual needs and activities later in life. The sculptor Michelangelo for example combined artistic with sexual prowess in his late sixties. The composer Haydn reached musical zenith in his late years while retaining his capacity for pleasure with the opposite sex. Even the Bible, with for example Sarah giving birth to Isaac when Abraham was a hundred years old, is quoted to show that previous societies did not try to condemn their elders to abstinence simply by reason of age. Critics of such examples can suggest that these examples are merely the exceptions which prove the rule. Doctors being scientific creatures will prefer evidence from old people themselves, for or against the idea.

I have mentioned in a previous chapter that many social and medical surveys of the elderly community have been carried out in the U.K., especially since 1948 (the start of the N.H.S.). Most of these have ignored sexual factors, apart from incidental inclusion when, say, measurements of sex hormones in the urine have been studied in connexion with longevity, or abnormalities with a sexual overtone have been recorded in cases of personality-change due to hardening of brain arteries. Studies from Holland, Sweden and the U.S.A. – many based on personal replies from questionnaire forms – are available and support the general assertion that sexual interest may be retained by both sexes late on in life.

Certain groups of doctors are more likely to come across sexual problems in middle and later age. Gynaecologists for example may be consulted because of loss of libido (or occasionally the opposite) in the woman passing or having just passed through the menopause. The psychiatrist also often has patients with this type of problem referred to him. Gynaecologists also see women in their sixties who complain of painful intercourse and are found to have a treatable physical condition locally, such as loss of the normal vaginal lining or a tiny overgrowth of urethral outlet at the vagina. Correction of this often brings much explicit thanks for restoring conjugal happiness.

Genito-urinary surgeons are familiar with the questions on sexual feelings and function which are asked by men, prior to operations on the genitals or prostate gland. Impotence is not invariable after such operations but may occur due to interruption of nerves. Today, with newer techniques that do not damage these nerves, impotence is more likely to be psychological in origin; that is, either the man expects to be impotent or he uses it as a convenient excuse for discontinuing already unwelcome sexual activity.

Similarly, the idea that womb removal (hysterectomy) or the change of life must be followed by loss of sexual desire in the female partner, is based on nothing more than a common emotional attitude. The lack of desire may be brought on by fear of unsuccessful or painful coitus, or the whole thing may represent a long-sought opportunity to terminate sexual relations and continue marriage on a basis of 'just good friends'.

Family doctors see patients who come complaining of

vague physical disabilities in their sixties, which on more intimate discussion reveal problems of a sexual nature. In the man, fear of waning sexual potency and ability to satisfy the needs of his wife, for example, may bring a direct question to the doctor either about giving up sexual relationship or about male hormones or aphrodisiacs. In the female, fears of waning attraction may again result in requests for hormone therapy or stimulants, or make her seek cosmetic help in the plastic surgeon's department.

The question of the disabilities of ageing interfering with regular sexual activity must arise. Heart and chest disease, limb disabilities and nervous system diseases may limit or entirely prevent one or other partner's active sexual participation. Even then, a mutually understanding couple with a good personal relationship may be able to enjoy limited sexual pleasure for a time.

Social workers, health visitors and geriatricians do come across sexual problems but are not ordinarily trained to counsel professionally on these matters. They may try to help on the basis of their own commonsense and background knowledge but may be unable to manipulate the environment or to influence the fixed emotional attitudes of wife or husband. Where these last are the obstacle, and in cases where organic brain disease leads to abnormal sexual desires or possibly anti-social action, professional psychiatric help is called for as with any other mental aberration.

That interest and genuine appreciation of the opposite sex is present in older people, is borne out by the marriages which stem from friendships in over-60s clubs or in welfare homes. Improvement in physical well-being and mental outlook in the ensuing generations of old people may reveal the truth about sex in the later years and may ultimately change the attitude of twentieth-century society towards it.

8

DRUG THERAPY FOR THE ELDERLY

APPROACH TO DRUG TREATMENT

THERE are certain principles of drug treatment which are universally applicable. The doctor examines his patient, after taking the medical history, and asks himself three basic questions. Firstly, does the patient actually need a drug? If a patient has suffered, for example, from irregularity or 'obstinate bowels' most of her life, she may ask the doctor for something to remedy the situation right away. Before hurrying to prescribe, say, senna or cascara, he might consider whether his patient takes enough fluid in each twenty-four hours, whether he or she eats enough bulking and roughage foods such as vegetables or fruit, and visits the W.C. whenever 'the call' comes, and whether, if the patient is up, more activity might help matters. On the other hand, he may reflect that this patient's bowel activity has depended on say, regular liquid paraffin or aloes for many years, and agree to his or her usual dose of laxative to relieve the situation.

Secondly, what form of the drug – solid, liquid or injection – should he use? For example, if a patient is unconscious, there is no use trying to get him or her to swallow syrup – injection into vein or muscle will be necessary. If the patient is conscious and cooperative, but has trouble swallowing large pills, the doctor may prescribe smaller pills or a liquid syrup or mixture. If the patient dislikes 'taking things' – 'they make me choke' or 'feel sick' – and injections are thought to be too painful, suppositories can be given, which are absorbed through the rectum.

Thirdly, the most important question of all, what is the smallest effective dose reliable and which can be given for the shortest possible time? In all age groups, this last point is important but in the elderly it is the most important of all, bar none.

PATTERN OF DRUG THERAPY

In two previous chapters, I have pointed out that elderly patients may be suffering from three to six illnesses or disabilities when first seen by the doctor. The diseases may be directly connected with each other, as for instance colds, bronchitis, pneumonia, heart failure and swelling of both legs, or they may be unrelated – say, cirrhosis of the liver, urinary infection, deafness, and weakness of the left arm and leg. Multiple diseases might appear to call for multiple drugs. But if all the patient's conditions are treated at once, he or she will complain 'I'm rattling' or, more seriously, be weakened, nauseated and depressed by this over-enthusiastic therapy. The doctor therefore singles out, as we have seen, the one or two illnesses which immediately threaten the patient's life, and he prescribes suitable drugs for these. At judicious periods in the recovering stage that follows, he drops the 'life-savers' and brings in any other drugs needed to complete the patient's return to the fullest health possible. Some conditions, particularly less urgent surgical procedures, e.g. for rupture or piles, are postponed for several months to allow for convalescence.

All drugs have some unwanted effects which are incidental to the main therapeutic effect of the drug. These unwanted or side-effects, such as, for example, dry mouth with artane therapy for parkinsonism, can be a nuisance, but worth putting up with for the main good result. The side-effects old people suffer are just like those for younger age groups, but they may be exaggerated, for three reasons: older patients

116

are more forgetful than younger ones and may either take two doses at once as a 'precaution' or take too many without realizing it; illness or ageing of the kidney and liver organs may result in failure to remove the drug quickly, causing poisonous accumulation and an 'overdose' effect; the 'target organ' affected by the drug, e.g. the heart, may be damaged so that the 'usually effective' dose is really too much and the effect too powerful. Phenobarbitone, frequently prescribed as a sedative for young people or for 'fits', is a good example: taking too many tablets can cause stupor or coma, failure of liver detoxication and failure of kidney excretion into the urine can cause 'build-up' in the bloodstream and again stupor or coma, while a 'stroke' that has affected the brain may allow even a quarter of a grain to have the effect of three grains, when again stupor or coma results.

TREATING THE CAUSE

From the earliest part of this book, I have stressed the importance of finding the cause of a disturbance in an old person and treating the cause, not just the symptoms. In old people, where confusion is the commonest symptom whatever the cause, this is even more important. For example there is no point in giving an old man nothing but heavy doses of a tranquilliser if his restlessness and confusion are due to the fever of a pneumonia. Penicillin or other antibiotic therapy to heal the pneumonia is basically more important. Of course, in a hospital ward with other sick or ill patients, or even at home where there are children off to school and menfolk off to work in the morning, night sedation of the pneumonia patient may be necessary. In that case, the smallest effective dose could be given with great caution provided antibiotics are already being administered, too, and on the understanding that it is a socio-medical compromise.

In a similar vein, the prescribing of vitamins for old

people should be based on definite evidence of deficiency based on examination of the patient or his regular (or irregular) diet. We have seen in the nutrition section, that malnutrition and imperfect diets may arise from physical illness, mental disturbance, lack of cooking knowledge or lack of finance. Under such circumstances, the administration of tablets or injections (for more rapid effect) of multi-vitamins – B,A,D,C and K – is well justified. Of course if overt scurvy or 'old people's rickets' or a tendency to bleed is present, the appropriate vitamin should be given alone in full therapeutic dose.

If, however, an old person is eating a full diet containing adequate quantities of vitamins, and comes complaining of vague aches and pains or general malaise, there is no point in giving large amounts of vitamin preparations just because the advertisers tell us how young they will keep us. Vitamin B12 deficiency, which causes pernicious anaemia and nervous system disturbances, is commoner in middle and old age than in young people. It can be corrected by regular injections of hydroxycobalamin which, once started, must be continued for the rest of the patient's life.

Pernicious anaemia is an example of a deficiency disease – that is, illness due to a missing chemical in the bloodstream. Such diseases as hypothyroidism (lack of thyroid), hypoadrenalism (lack of steroid hormones from the suprarenal glands), sugar diabetes (lack of body-produced insulin) of the more severe type are all deficiency illnesses treated by replacement of the missing chemical – thyroid, cortisone and insulin in the above examples. In old people with such illnesses, the problem is to ensure that they continue taking this replacement therapy for the rest of their days. If they feel well again, it is sometimes hard to persuade them that they are not 'cured', merely kept on an even keel by the chemical. Moreover, forgetting or taking the wrong dose because of slow thought or poor memory can result in relapse – this applies to all old persons who have to take drugs, whether for replacement or other therapy. In the case of injection treatment, like daily insulin or fortnightly hydroxycobalamin, the district nurse may visit the old person regularly to ensure the right treatment. In the case of tablets, relatives, neighbours or friends may be delegated to ensure regular correct therapy.

DRUGS AGAINST AGEING

The most important problems in geriatrics stem from two major pathological changes in the body – hardening of the arteries, called atherosclerosis, and malignant change in tissues or organs, called cancer.

Atherosclerosis particularly affects the arteries of brain, heart and limbs, with secondary effects from the diminished blood and oxygen supply to end organs. Claims have been made that drugs which could open up or widen the arteries – vasodilators – would counter the effects of artery hardening and poor blood supply. Unfortunately, while healthy arteries do expand with these drugs, narrowed and hardened arteries do so little or not at all, and vasodilators have proved disappointing in atherosclerosis. The use of cholesterol–fatty acid lowering agents, both drugs and vegetable oils, has been shown experimentally to slow up atherosclerosis in the animal, but the results in humans are not fully conclusive; nor do the drugs definitely reverse any atherosclerosis already established in the elderly patient.

From time to time, our press reports startling new treatments to slow up or reverse the ageing process in men and women. Closer examination of such reports usually reveals that the 'foreign clinic' or 'sex specialist' treatments are based on the giving of sex hormones, a procedure which is far from new. There are certain clear indications for giving sex hormones or their chemical relatives to people; for example, as I mentioned above, steroids in suprarenal deficiency, or anabolic male hormone to build up thin bones or muscle in a malnourished or post-operative patient. Neither the latter male hormones or the female oestrogens can truthfully be described as anti-ageing, even though they may partially counteract tissue changes such as muscle thinning or skin texture. There is no hormone 'elixir of life', and the effects of any 'rejuvenation treatment' are often largely psychological, the 'patient' feeling better but medically really in no different case.

In the case of malignant disease, progress has been steady. Encouraging old (and younger) people to report to their own doctor anything unusual – for instance (in women) a lump in the breast or minor but unexpected bleeding from the vaginal orifice, or (in men) a persistent cough or difficulties with passing urine – often means earlier diagnosis and a better chance of successful treatment. The four bulwarks of therapy against cancer are surgical removal, radiation therapy, hormone therapy and anti-cancer-cell drugs. Any of these may be combined to give a better result in a given case. Surgical operations are no longer excluded merely on the grounds of age. Better and safer anaesthetics, quicker and more efficient operative techniques, careful pre-operative assessment and building-up and careful attention to chest, excretory function and pressure areas after an operation, have greatly improved an old person's chances.

PLACEBO THERAPY

The placebo is a tablet or a mixture or even an injection, which has no chemical effect that is therapeutic, but is given to a patient as a psychological bolster. In the days, not so very long ago, when effective drugs for physical illnesses and for anxiety states, insomnia, neuroses or 'nervous breakdowns' were not always available, administration of an inert substance, coloured say red or blue or with a distinctive taste, and accompanied by reassurance, was a perfectly rational therapy. Today, however, the advances in chemical therapy for all varieties of physical and mental illness – from minor to major – means that there are effective sedatives, hypnotics, tranquillizers, analgesics and antibiotics, for example, available to treat them. The use of the placebo is therefore not justified, and least of all with elderly people, where symptoms of, say, confusion and restlessness, in the old days 'classics' for placebo-type prescriptions, so often spring from physical disorders that may be treatable once diagnosed (see pages 45–6). The only occasion which requires such a fake or spoof drug is a 'drug trial' where a new drug is compared with a similar looking 'blank' tablet to test whether it is the patient's mind or the actual chemical that is 'curing' the condition.

THE FUTURE OF GERIATRICS

ONE SPECIALTY OR SEVERAL?

THE specialty of paediatric medicine – treatment of diseases of childhood – grew out of the realization that medically speaking, children were not mini-adults. First, the question of doses of drugs given to infants and children was shown to be not one of percentage dosage but of treating children as a separate medical group. Secondly, it became obvious that disease incidence and disease patterns in children were different from those in adults. Thirdly, it was realized that social factors – environment, intelligence of parents, social class – were greatly influential in the progress of children who were ill and in the prevention of disease in infancy and childhood. Paediatrics gradually appeared as a separate subject for study in the medical student's curriculum and gradually all medical schools throughout Great Britain appointed professors in paediatric medicine and sick children's hospitals came into their own.

The parallel with geriatrics is striking. As we have seen in previous chapters, the general pattern of dosage and drug therapy for adults has to be modified for elderly people. Disease incidence and disease pattern are also different in the elderly, with degenerative disease and malignant disease playing still greater roles. Social factors – living alone or otherwise, age of relatives, income – greatly influence the progress and outcome of illness in old people. Preventive geriatrics, too, is analogous to preventive techniques of immunization, screening and biochemical assessment of infants and children.

The question then arises whether geriatrics in the future will like paediatrics develop its own internal specialties – as surgical paediatrics, orthopaedic paediatrics, child psychiatry, so operative geriatrics, orthogeriatrics, and psychogeriatrics. Many geriatrics specialists admit that one of the fascinations of practising their specialty is the broad base of medicine, surgery, physical medicine, psychological medicine and surgical knowledge which is required. This allows an all-round approach to the patient and prevents the 'case of such-and-such disease' classification clouding the issue. It may be, however, that some specialists in other fields, genitourinary surgeons, for instance, or gynaecologists, will take a greater interest in geriatrics and regard themselves as 'branch geriatricians'. It is also true that individual geriatricians already take a special interest in conditions such as, say, thyroid disease or valvular heart disease or arthritic disease, on which they have done research work and in which they develop an expertise.

TEACHING UNITS IN GERIATRICS

At the time of writing, there is still only one professorial chair in geriatric medicine, that of Professor Anderson at the University of Glasgow. It is hoped that other university centres will follow suit and establish chairs and attached departments. When I was an undergraduate more than a decade ago, the subject of geriatrics was tackled in one lecture under the 'Public Health' heading; the rest was up to the individual medical student and, later, to the doctor in practice. Today, and certainly tomorrow, undergraduate study of the social and medical problems of the elderly is a must for the trainee doctor, whatever path he intends to take after qualification.

The absence of official teaching units has not prevented, as we have seen, the growth and flowering of this specialty of treating the elderly patient. All geriatricians regard it as a duty if not a real pleasure to teach medical students, doctors and nurses the principles and practice of geriatrics, much of which I have outlined in preceding chapters. Hospital libraries are encouraged to carry the many books and journals which are devoted to geriatrics on both sides of the Atlantic. At one time, doctors who wanted 'plenty of time to study' and little 'work to do on the wards' took house doctor or senior house doctor posts in geriatrics. These junior doctors often found that they had stumbled on a busy, rewarding post with a wealth of clinical interest and a need to apply all their previous training in the broadest manner for the best results. Recruitment, personally or by clinical contact, has led these same doctors on to the senior grades of geriatrics or made them more effective and more interested family doctors in practice.

Of course, bona fide geriatric teaching units ought to have links with the university, which will encourage parallel research work in the problems and diseases of old age. Such research would stimulate more clinical effort and improve the services to the old at home and in hospital. Geriatricians ought to be able to travel abroad for research work on a much bigger scale than at present, so widening the individual's horizon and ensuring that international advances are available to all old people on a world-wide basis.

PREVENTION IS BETTER THAN CURE

While old age is not in itself a disease (and no 'cure' for healthy old age is likely), the value of preventive work in geriatrics has already been stressed. The preventive health clinic and the family doctor health centre are structural mainstays and the health visitor, family doctor and geriatrician complete the scaffolding on which old people can build a healthier old age. Mass screening surveys for malignant disease, sugar diabetes, vitamin deficiency or tuberculosis, for example, can be carried out on a community basis. Research work by physiologists and biochemists on the causes of hardening of the arteries and cancerous illnesses, and diets, drugs or patterns of life that can modify or prevent them, are all in progress, and better treatment and therapies for the established illnesses are on the way.

The antibiotics, substitute drugs like insulin, vaccines like those which protect against polio and smallpox, effective drugs for irregular and failing hearts, all have improved the outlook for the ill young adult and ill old person, and early diagnosis with early administration can prevent deterioration and cure bacterial infections at least. There is no reason to suppose that further advances along these lines will be any less rewarding and probably they will be even more successful.

The prevention of trauma for or injury to old people is being recognized as of increasing importance. Accidents in the home, for example, are a major cause of broken limbs, concussion, and the need for hospital admission to surgical or orthopaedic wards. All members of the geriatric team and voluntary and professional workers 'in the field' can guide and advise old people on the dangers of carpeting or rugs which are not nailed down, or split-level floors with badly lit steps, or polished linoleum floors, or household needs kept on high shelves, for example. They can check that the gas cooker is not likely to be left on and arrange through the Gas Board that the forgetful or partially-sighted or people with a poor sense of smell have automatic or safety lighting cookers. Future accommodation for the elderly should incorporate all such safety precautions, together with suitable heating, such as underfloor or central, suitable wall handrails and double rails on steps, and bells or light or Tannoy systems for emergency calls to wardens or other helpers.

On the road, children and old people suffer the highest

casualty rate. Patrolled crossings appear to be safest for old people – lighted crossings with elaborate 'go–don't go' flashing lights are less satisfactory. Interestingly, the 'lollipop' men and women who control children's crossing to and from school are frequently in the over-65 age group, and can be very efficient if in good health, for the short periods this job entails.

Deafness, poor vision and slower responses make people in their seventies and eighties very vulnerable to the density and high speeds of today's traffic. Fortunately, most people have a strong sense of duty about ushering elderly people across roads and they do not usually have to wait till a policeman or boy scout appears. In hospital, newer techniques for treating broken limbs by pinning and plating of the fractures, means earlier mobilization and return to community life for those who do become casualties.

DIFFERENCES IN DISEASE PATTERN

The frequent presence of multiple illness in the sick elderly has been stressed several times. What has not been mentioned until this chapter, is the altered pattern familiar adult diseases take on when they occur in old age. As study of the elderly goes on in clinical and laboratory work, the reasons for these differences in signs and symptoms will emerge. Meanwhile physicians specializing in treatment in old age are alive to the different clinical features a disease may present (including failure to present some 'classical' ones) at this stage of life.

For example, a clot in a major artery to the heart – coronary thrombosis – in a younger person produces severe crushing pains in the chest behind the breastbone, often passing up to the jaws or down the left arm. It is accompanied by a state of shock with cold sweating, clamminess, pale skin, a rapid thready pulse and a falling blood pressure. The symptoms are so dramatic that urgent medical attention is sought and often rapid admission to hospital forthcoming. In the elderly individual, a vague discomfort, often thought to be indigestion, replaces the classical crushing pain. A feeling of weakness or being 'a little off-colour' replaces the classical shock. The first real sign of a serious heart attack may, indeed, be a stroke or paralysis affecting one side of the body, due to the falling blood pressure. It may be only when an electrocardiogram of the old person is taken, that the true illness comes to light.

Sugar diabetes is another complaint that has a distinctive pattern, as a rule, in elderly persons. As already briefly mentioned, obesity in old people is significantly associated with diabetes. The weight gain seems to produce stress on the old person's pancreas, reducing the body's output of insulin into the bloodstream. Whereas in young diabetics, injection of insulin daily is called for, in the old person, a weight-reducing diet that is later adjusted to maintain an 'ideal' weight for height and age, will often alone control the sugar diabetes. In some cases, however, drugs like the sulphonylureas are added to the diet to encourage the body to release more insulin and control the sugar. Occasionally elderly people have a severe diabetes that is not controllable by diet or drugs and needs insulin. This may call for regular visits by the district nurse to ensure correct dosage and by the health visitor to ensure a proper diet. Further investigation into the causes of sugar diabetes may reveal why the illness is usually milder in the elderly than in young people.

Another example is the condition of peritonitis, due for example to rupture of an acutely inflamed appendix. In the young adult, the onset shows the classical features of pain in the centre of the abdomen with sickness and vomiting, the pain later moving to the lower right side of the abdomen. There is slight fever and marked local tenderness on touching this lower right area. In the elderly person, there may be no history of real pain or only a vague generalized discomfort, no sickness or perhaps very mild nausea and no really localized tender area in the abdomen. The temperature may or may not go up and all one really observes is an old person 'below par' with a vague 'stomach upset'. As the peritonitis progresses in the young person, he becomes cold, clammy, sweating and shocked, with a rigid tender abdomen, and is in great danger unless treated. Our old patient may still have only vague signs at this stage though obviously 'going downhill'.

In the case of heart disease due to gradual hardening of the arteries, patients in old age rarely complain of tightening chest pain on effort like going up slopes or steps (the angina of younger people) but only of vague 'weakness' or of 'feeling done'. Again such remarks must not just be attributed to their 'not being as young as they were'. What is called 'ischaemic heart disease' must be looked for and excluded, or confirmed as a diagnosis for treatment.

The importance of appreciating the 'milder appearance' of many serious illnesses in the elderly is well known to geriatricians and this knowledge can be passed on to other doctors in training or in practice.

The increased tendency of old people to develop growths or tumours has also been mentioned. Various explanations have been suggested for this, but the actual process will probably be determined in the general research on the causes of cancer and malignant blood diseases. Fortunately, however, the running down or thinning of some tissues in old people has a protective role, in slowing up any abnormal tumours growing in an organ. The growth of malignant cells is known to be dependent on a good blood supply, bringing plenty of glucose and protein. Where 'ageing' has replaced working cells with scar tissue and where hardened arteries have reduced blood flow to an organ, tumours find it harder to grow. In fact older patients may, as it were, outlive their growths and die from some other, unrelated illness.

OTHER POINTS OF ADVANCE

One particular illness which is frequently missed by doctors and nurses attending an old person is myxoedema, caused by failure of the thyroid gland to produce the hormone, thyroxine. The features of myxoedema – thinning hair and eyebrows, loss of skin elasticity with wrinkling and puffiness round the eyes, intolerance of cold weather, deafness, slowness of thought and movement, constipation – all these are 'classically' associated with ageing. However, certain signs will suggest the illness to the specialist, who can do two blood tests to confirm or rule out thyroid deficiency. Myxoedema will respond slowly but surely to the giving of thyroid tablets, which are cautiously increased in dose over a few weeks so as not to upset the old person's heart. After three months, the old person may be blessing the physician for new life and a revitalized appearance: photographs taken 'before and after' are often the most convincing evidence of the change. In the future, prevention of myxoedema may be possible when we know and can interrupt the factors which 'damp down' the thyroid gland or permanently damage its working.

Disturbances in the regular blood supply to the brain are commoner in old people than among adults generally, usually resulting from hardening of the arteries or high blood pressure or a combination of these. The symptoms may range from mild giddiness or unsteadiness on looking up or walking, through feelings of faintness or, occasionally, blackouts, to sudden or gradual onset of weakness or paralysis in the limbs of one side. Much research is going on into the dynamics of brain circulation and whether these can be altered or improved by drugs or surgery. In the meantime, encouragement, suitable exercises, aids to walking and steadiness like

frames and walking sticks, short inpatient treatment in rehabilitation wards or longer inpatient treatment in the case
of more severe paralysis, are practical steps in the therapy of
such disturbance.

Diseases affecting the joints are common in the elderly.
The 'wear and tear' osteoarthritis affects weight-bearing
joints like hips and knees and, as we noted earlier, is made
worse by obesity. Rheumatoid arthritis, an allergic type of
joint disease once thought to occur only in young people,
is now known to occur in the 60s and 70s. Research
into rheumatoid arthritis should be showing results. In the
meantime, although roughly one new drug has been discovered every three years since the late 1950s claiming to be
the most effective in relieving pain and damping down inflammation in this illness (which affects hands, wrists, ankles
and feet), aspirin remains the basis of most antirheumatic
therapy. Aspirin is also effective in relieving the discomfort
of osteoarthritis. Elderly patients with painful stiff joints
have a tendency to take to bed sooner than younger housewives or working people with the same illness. Locking of
joints in bent, awkward positions may call for admission to
the rehabilitation ward when the inflammation has subsided.
There, heat, exercises for weak and wasted muscles, splints
and plasters, can be used to correct deformities and make the
patient mobile again with frame, crutches or a walking stick.
I have personally seen a set of three patients, bed-bound for
nine, six and five years respectively, being enabled to walk
under their own steam. Of course, the sooner treatment is
begun the better and I am not recommending years of bed
care as a good preliminary . . .

Sometimes old people act as a source of infection without
being aware that they are really ill and passing on infection to
younger people. Tuberculosis, for example, may be masked
in the elderly by chronic bronchitis; 'granpa is in and out of
bed, has a lot of cough and phlegm and is thin and under-

weight', relatives may register, with no one realizing he has chronic fibrotic tuberculosis until a grandchild develops fluid in the chest, or a daughter-in-law with whom he lives gets night sweats, a cough, starts wasting and is found to have active lung tuberculosis. Fortunately this is uncommon and even less likely in the present era of regular check-ups and preventive clinics.

A PSYCHOGERIATRIC WARD

Professional and lay people are well aware of the mental disabilities and disturbances that are present in some old people. It might be thought superfluous therefore to coin the term 'psychogeriatrics', as if to denote a new entity in treatment of diseases of old age. Where the term is used, and where it is applied to a hospital ward, this should be only to clarify a situation or pinpoint a service provided for a particular patient, or group. It has already been pointed out that even if mental disturbances in ageing call for special services in a hospital, this should not prevent the doctor and his 'team' considering the patient's physical and social problems.

Most areas, as already explained, have access to geriatric units nowadays, and to these patients suffering temporary confusion can be sent. The building of local authority mental hostels for elderly people showing a more permanent mental change has begun in some areas, and should be taken up by other progressive local authorities in the future. Such hostels have been authorized by the Mental Health Act, 1959, for the psychiatric elderly requiring care but not active treatment. Elderly people with a mental illness such as depression with suicidal tendencies, can continue to go to mental hospitals for treatment in the usual way.

In the case of the second group – elderly people showing more lasting mental change in mental hostels – it would seem logical that if they require active treatment, this should be in a short-stay ward for a suitable period. When no longer needing active treatment, they could return to the mental hostel. This short-stay ward could be the basic concept for a 'psychogeriatric ward', but owing to the lack of mental welfare hostel places and the low 'turnover' in those already filled, the short-stay psychogeriatric ward might unwillingly become a long-stay ward.

An alternative type of psychogeriatric ward that may appear in general hospitals of the future, would be a 'first-entry confusion assessment' ward; where psychiatrist and geriatrician could work out jointly, after both had examined the patient, a coordinated individual plan of progress. A pilot unit of this type was established in Edinburgh in 1960, and results after a five-year period showed a 50 per cent discharge rate – to home, hostel or lodgings – but with difficulties arising from inadequate or insufficient home and hospital services and welfare accommodation. Such psychogeriatric assessment units could ensure that each patient was placed in the right setting for the right sort of therapy to give the best results.

AREA COORDINATOR OF GERIATRIC SERVICES?

In the early days of the National Health Service, hospital physicians watched with mixed feelings the disappearance of the medical superintendent post in hospital. Some felt that the transfer of medical administrative duties to group or hospital secretary or administrative clerical men would lead to difficulties. Problems in coordination, loss of efficiency and slowing of progressive policies through a lack of understanding of medical concepts and precepts, were forecast. Others welcomed the elimination of a post whose occupant might arrogate monarchical powers and unassailable influence in medical, nursing and administrative matters.

Astute observers saw that the governmental influence on the future of hospitals would call for a 'hospital civil service' led by trained professional lay administrators – whose minds were untrammelled by five or six years study of diseases, patients and their treatment.

Thus, superintendents retired and were not replaced and fond memories of old Mac or old Walrus-face faded gently into the past. The mental hospitals still retained the post, however, and the many Regional Boards, trying to keep up with the lay administrative Joneses, expanded their senior administrative *medical* officer grades with deputies and assistants.

The pundits who forecast disturbed hospital communications were much justified. Mixed lay and medical hospital management committees and associated area medical advisory committees produced that delight of democratic decisions – hospital red tape, and on a bigger scale than ever. Where one man had previously made an early and effective decision based on person-to-person communication, minutes and memos ricocheted between committees for months on end. When a decision was eventually made, it was either too late or too early for a given year's budget or turned down by the Regional Board. The pattern persists in hospitals all over the country, despite valiant personal efforts to streamline committees, speed up inter-communication and obviate delays.

The same criticism is often applied to the geriatric field. We have surveyed briefly the many different groups, professional, lay or voluntary, of people with a close interest in the present and future of the elderly. There are a number of central organizing bodies in each group but, especially in the hospital–Public Health sector, autonomous decisions are still very much the order of the day. The idea of a central authoritative figure who could 'overrule' decisions of different departments or groups may sound dictatorial, and doctors would be the first to agree that they are far from omniscient, but the consultant geriatrician is well-placed to play the role of area coordinator in geriatric services. Whether the institution of such a medical post could finally solve the representation and coordination problems of geriatric practice would have to be seen.

HOLIDAY RELIEF AND TERMINAL CARE

I have mentioned previously that most old people in the general community will be dependent on someone or some group after the age of 80. Also, I have noted that many even severely disabled old people are cared for by kind and willing relatives who do not complain and often forgo the pleasures of 'a night out' or 'a day at the seaside' or a proper holiday. This sort of situation may continue for many years. Geriatric units and welfare departments of the local authority consider that such relatives do deserve a holiday or temporary 'break' from attending their elderly charges. A few relatives may be able to afford the fees for a private nursing home for a period to give themselves a short holiday, and know that their old people are being nursed under supervision. Most are unable to find such fees and for these 'holiday relief' schemes in the summer months – when, in theory, pressure on geriatric beds and welfare homes places is lower – have been introduced. Usually for one or two weeks, with the heaviest intake at the local holiday period, bed or chair cases go to geriatric units and chair or ambulant cases to welfare homes. Relatives are asked to fit in with 'Saturday to Saturday' dates so that comings and goings dovetail.

Such holiday relief schemes again help to 'keep elderly patients at home' and have grown in scope over the country. Nevertheless they put a heavy load on the medical and nursing staff, since such admissions go on while staff is depleted by summer holiday rotas, and the rate of admissions to the unit – always high – suddenly quadruples. Also if the waiting list for 'regular' cases has grown and is still being vigorously reduced after the winter 'block', normal admission of ill and needy cases is likely to suffer, albeit temporarily. It may be, in the future, that specific hospital beds not actually in the geriatric unit establishment will be made available by the Boards and hospital management committees in each region, with temporary staff called in to nurse and doctor these 'relief cases' for the midsummer period. Alternatively, a given geriatric unit may have a small number of beds designated as 'holiday relief only' for all-year-round help to relatives, but the latter will then simply have to accept their break when the hospital gives the signal, not specify when they wish to take a 'holiday'.

Patients suffering from malignant disease which is beyond medical or surgical treatment so that they have only a few weeks or months to live – or other medical conditions which will result in early death – such patients still need good nursing care with attention to nutrition, hygiene and the relief of pain or discomfort. Again, many relatives take on this care – of young or old terminal cases – with great determination and courage, and are well supported by their family doctor and district nurse and other services. However some patients require hospital-type nursing at an early or late stage. In the days before official geriatric units, the usual pattern was for the unit which had treated the patient originally, e.g. medical or surgical, to readmit him or her to the ward for the last period of the illness. In fact, some hospital units still do things this way. Many doctors and specialists say, however, that as geriatric units are responsible for 'chronic sick' (now long-stay) beds, such units are the logical place for all terminal care patients.

There appears to be no 'official' policy for the care of such unfortunate patients. Geriatric units do take their share – sometimes the lion's share – of terminal cases, but dislike it when young patients, say women with inoperable cancer of the womb in their thirties, are referred to them and have to see out their days in the company of elderly disabled or frail people. The Marie Curie Foundation has established suitable nursing homes for the terminal care of cancer patients in several areas. In the future, a proper policy for non-geriatric long-stay cases (and young people also come under this heading who are not terminally ill but require long-term nursing for disabilities) will have to be worked out by the Ministry of Health and the various interested parties.

ENVOI

TALKING to a luncheon club recently, I suggested that the rights of old age could be thought of in terms of the late President F. D. Roosevelt's famous four freedoms – freedom of speech and expression, freedom to worship God in one's own way, freedom from fear and freedom from want. In the light of my own and others' experience, I suggested two further freedoms – freedom from unnecessary ill-health and freedom from undue dependence.

We have been concerned with some of these freedoms in the various chapters of this short book. Freedom of speech and expression is not always available to an old person. This may be the result of being alone and not in contact with daily life, or it may be that, while living with relatives, he or she is not allowed to play a verbal role in the family's life. Brain disturbances from hardening of the arteries, or a 'stroke', or just ill-fitting dentures may produce distortion of speech physically. Younger companions or visitors note the old person's remarkable memory for distant or past events, but tendency to forget the most recent happenings; and may act impatient with a habit of repeating the same story over and over again. (Not that that habit is an old people's monopoly.)

Freedom of worship exists in this country. British people have a broad tolerance of all creeds and religions. We have to remember, though, that old people must often depend on others to let them exercise their right to formal observance and contact with fellow-believers. Those confined to their homes depend on the visiting parson or priest. Most ministers of religion are conscientious about seeing to their non-mobile parishioners. In hospital, every effort is made to ensure that the ministers can see members of their own faith and be available at times of stress or when life is ebbing. (Young people sometimes criticize their elders for their remarkable faith and strong religious interest. I have heard the unpleasant sneer that such godliness stems from their closeness to the final hour and the need to make amends for ill behaviour or wickedness. Perhaps this is only a reflection of a social climate which negates religion or relegates it to a minor role.)

Freedom from want, as we saw in the chapter on the socio-economic aspect of geriatrics, has not been attained. I have made some suggestions that would help to improve matters and hope that for the future newer income-related schemes for retirement benefits will successfully solve this problem in terms of hard cash. I find it ironical that television, which is often such a boon to housebound or lonely old people, should flaunt the latest, greatest, newest good things of the material life at their current prices to someone with £4 a week to live on.

Freedom from fear can be subdivided for the elderly into freedom from fear of being lonely and freedom from fear of approaching death. Loneliness, as we have noted, is the factor which voluntary workers and groups work hardest at combating. Poverty, changes in family life, changing accommodation, are all factors that can entail this for the elderly, and the value of clubs and centres has been stressed. Fear of approaching death strikes all of us at some time or other when we leave childhood and realize that after all we are not immortal. The loss of contemporaries and loved ones brings the point home over the years. Some people will inevitably equate old age with death and so attempt to shut out the advancing years. Others will be just as busy and interested in the surrounding world at 80 as they were thirty years before. Most old people face the coming departure with remarkable equanimity, especially if they have left their 'mark' through their grandchildren, or through some artistic or literary or professional success.

Freedom from unnecessary ill-health has been dealt with under the preventive geriatrics heading. It is what is being striven for in the whole approach of modern geriatric assessment and rehabilitation, backing the family doctor's attention. Old age by itself is not a disease or an excuse for doing nothing. Freedom from undue dependence must vary with the physical and mental health of each old person and these in turn with the interest of the attendants on the old person and the stimulus they offer. Initiative should always be encouraged at every stage of recovery from an illness.

It may be that professional and voluntary workers in geriatrics, and relatives and friends of old people, will read this short book and accuse me of painting too rosy a picture of geriatrics today. They might tell me that I have glossed over the unpleasant aspects of nursing an aged incontinent patient or trying to cope with a confused relative in a busy working household. If so, I admit that I have tried to spread optimism, and a forward-looking approach, in most of the chapters and to warn against the lethargic attitude that bedevilled old age in the past. Difficulties and problems abound, and will have to be vigorously tackled along the way, but if the goal is a fuller, healthier and happier old age, only the most hopeful footsteps will ensure our eventual arrival.

INDEX

MORE ABOUT PENGUINS
AND PELICANS

Penguin Book News, which appears every month, contains details of all the new books issued by Penguins as they are published. From time to time it is supplemented by *Penguins in Print* – a complete list of all our available titles. (There are well over three thousand of these.)

A specimen copy of *Penguin Book News* will be sent to you free on request and you can become a subscriber for the price of the postage – 4s for a year's issues (including the complete lists). Just write to Dept EP, Penguin Books Ltd, Harmondsworth, Middlesex, enclosing a cheque or postal order, and your name will be added to the mailing list.

Another Pelican is described overleaf.

Note: *Penguin Book News* and *Penguins in Print* are not available in the U.S.A. or Canada

THE PSYCHOLOGY OF
HUMAN AGEING

D. B. Bromley

Infant and adolescent psychology have been very thoroughly explored: but the study of ageing lags behind.

A gerontologist, who is scientific adviser in this field to the Medical Research Council, fills a gap in the literature of psychology with this new introduction to human ageing and its mental effects. Dealing with the course of life from maturity onwards, Dr Bromley examines many biological and social effects of human ageing; personality and adjustment; mental disorders in adult life and old age; age changes in the organization of occupational and skilled performance; adult intelligence; and age changes in intellectual, social, and other achievements. A final section on method in the study of ageing makes this book an important contribution for the student of psychology as well as the layman.